OBAMACARE WARS

Studies in Government
and Public Policy

OBAMACARE WARS

Federalism, State Politics, and the Affordable Care Act

Daniel Béland, Philip Rocco, and Alex Waddan

 University Press of Kansas

Published by the University Press of Kansas (Lawrence, Kansas 66045), which was organized by the Kansas Board of Regents and is operated and funded by Emporia State University, Fort Hays State University, Kansas State University, Pittsburg State University, the University of Kansas, and Wichita State University

Library of Congress Cataloging-in-Publication Data
Names: Béland, Daniel. | Rocco, Philip. | Waddan, Alex, 1964–
Title: Obamacare wars : federalism, state politics, and the affordable care act /
Daniel Béland, Philip Rocco, and Alex Waddan.
Description: Lawrence, Kansas : University Press of Kansas, [2016] |
Series: Studies in government and public policy |
Includes bibliographical references and index.
Identifiers: LCCN 2015032190 | ISBN 9780700621910 (cloth : alk. paper) |
    ISBN 9780700635078 (paperback : alk. paper) | ISBN 9780700621965 (ebook)
Subjects: LCSH: Health care reform—United States. | Medical policy—United States. |
    Medical care—United States.
Classification: LCC RA395.D44 B45 2016 | DDC 368.38/200973—dc23 LC record
    available at http://lccn.loc.gov/2015032190.

British Library Cataloguing-in-Publication Data is available.

Printed in the United States of America

10 9 8 7 6 5 4 3 2 1

The paper used in this publication is acid free and meets the minimum requirements of the American National Standard for Permanence of Paper for Printed Library Materials Z39.48-1992.

CONTENTS

TABLES

FIGURES

ACRONYMS

ACA   Patient Protection and Affordable Care Act

AHIP   America's Health Insurance Providers

ALEC   American Legislative Exchange Council

CCIIO   Center for Consumer Information and Insurance Oversight

CHIP   Children's Health Insurance Program

CMS   Centers for Medicare and Medicaid Services

HIPAA   Health Insurance Portability and Accountability Act

HHS   Department of Health and Human Services

MLR   medical loss ratio

NAIC   National Association of Insurance Commissioners

NAMD   National Association of Medicaid Directors

NFIB   National Federation of Independent Business

PREFACE TO THE PAPERBACK EDITION

When the COVID-19 pandemic hit, Louise Snodgrass was worried. Despite experiencing COVID-like symptoms on several occasions, the twenty-six-year-old farmers market manager from Brookings, South Dakota, without health insurance did not get tested for the virus and never went to the doctor. Even after enrolling in an insurance plan through the Patient Protection and Affordable Care Act (ACA)'s federal exchange in January 2021, Snodgrass found that the monthly premiums and $6,000 deductible still put needed care out of reach. But there was no other viable option. Unlike most state governments, South Dakota had not yet implemented the ACA's Medicaid expansion. Nearly two years later, in November 2022, the state's voters approved a ballot measure calling for the expansion to be implemented in the state, although there was no immediate date set for when that would happen.[1]

Six years after we first published *Obamacare Wars*, more than a decade after the ACA became law and amid a pandemic, federalism continues to shape the contours of healthcare policy and politics in the United States. Even as the ACA drastically reduced the number of Americans without health insurance—the uninsured rate among the nonelderly population fell from 18 percent in 2010 to a little over 10 percent by the end of the decade—there is still substantial variation across states. In 2020, the rate of nonelderly persons without health insurance ranged from 2.8 percent in Massachusetts to 20 percent in Texas.[2] These highly variable policy trajectories have significant impacts in state health outcomes. As a national study published in 2017 suggests, Medicaid expansion is responsible for saving one life annually for every 239–316 adults gaining insurance.[3]

To better understand the ACA's divergent policy trajectories, *Obamacare Wars* focuses on how the design of the ACA and its interaction with preexisting policy and political dynamics in the states affected its implementation. When major legislation is signed into law, it is not the end of the policy process but rather the beginning of the postreform political contest over its implementation, which is a crucial moment that can have durable consequences for the long-term fate of the reform at hand.[4] In a federal country like the United States, postreform politics is likely to prove especially contentious when states play a direct role in the implementation of (and sometimes even veto) key aspects of the enacted reform. This is particularly the case in an era of exacerbated partisanship when collaboration between Democrats and Republicans has become increasingly difficult and point-scoring and party victories trump more meaningful policy considerations.[5]

The hardcover edition of *Obamacare Wars*, which appeared in early 2016, covered the period from March 2010 to the end of the first open-enrollment period on the ACA's insurance marketplaces in late March 2014. Much has happened since then. Yet, more than six years after the publication of the book, we remain convinced that our analysis offers key insights about the politics of ACA implementation in the fifty states and in the broader context of US federalism. In this preface to the paperback edition, we will return to our main claims before discussing how the politics of ACA implementation has evolved since 2014 and, finally, we will offer some thoughts about how our book continues to remain relevant to the study of ACA politics specifically and US federalism more generally.[6]

Because of the ACA's complexity, we decided to focus on three main aspects of the legislation that involve a direct role for the states: health insurance exchanges, the expansion of Medicaid, and regulatory reform. First, the process of setting up health insurance exchanges to help businesses and families buy insurance was a major aspect of the ACA. The legislation charged the states with the responsibility to create these exchanges, yet a default provision allowed the federal government to step in and implement these if states failed to act. The second aspect of the ACA we address, the expansion of Medicaid to support people with income up to 138 percent of the federal poverty rate, differed from health insurance exchanges in that it could only take place with the support of each state government, even if the federal government agreed to cover a large portion of the costs. Finally, regulatory reform, in contrast to both the implementation of the exchanges and of Medicaid expansion, mainly featured low-profile bureaucratic policymaking that made for a less contentious policy arena and was characterized by greater levels of cooperation and consent. This was the case in part because regulatory reform involved much less partisan grandstanding than the exchanges and Medicaid expansion—two arenas in which many Republican policymakers who held political control of their states expressed their opposition to the ACA in a performative and even theatrical manner. Our analysis suggests that the creation of health insurance exchanges proved to be the most contentious site of postreform politics, more so than Medicaid expansion and regulatory reform. To explain variations among these three case studies, *Obamacare Wars* stresses the interaction among three main factors: policy legacies, institutional fragmentation, and public sentiments. We argue that these forces, when taken together, significantly shape the opportunities for dissent and consent among state policymakers.

In the years since we published *Obamacare Wars*, the election of Donald Trump and the brief period of unified Republican government in Washington (2017–2018) appeared to threaten the implementation and even the very existence of the ACA. Yet the net impact of these threats was far more limited than the law's supporters initially feared. First, Republicans could not easily make good on their efforts to "repeal and replace" the law through the legislative process. Captured by intense, ideologically motivated policy demanders, the Republican Party was only able to advance alternatives to the ACA that would raise insurance premiums and increase the size of the uninsured population and were thus deeply unpopular. This helped to both galvanize the loose constituencies of the ACA's supporters and internally divide congressional Republicans. By the end of 2017, Congress had only succeeded in eliminating the tax penalties imposed by the individual mandate, a feat that was only achieved by rolling the repeal into a $1.5 trillion tax cut package.[7] Where public opinion was concerned, the legislative effort to repeal and replace the ACA did little to mobilize the Republican base but instead helped to strengthen support for the law across the political spectrum.[8]

Efforts to gut the ACA through federal litigation also bore little fruit. As the framers of the ACA anticipated, a majority of states did not set up their own health insurance exchange. Instead, these states relied on the ACA's default provision for the federal government to run the insurance marketplace. This in turn formed the basis of King v. Burwell, a legal challenge to the ACA heard by the Supreme Court in early 2015. Here, the plaintiffs insisted that the language of the ACA meant that the Internal Revenue Service was only authorized to provide tax credits to people buying insurance through an exchange run by the states, not the federal government. One study estimated that if the plaintiffs were successful, 8.2 million people would lose their insurance.[9] In an op-ed in the New England Journal of Medicine, a trio of experienced health policy commentators warned that "ACA supporters . . . have good reason to worry."[10] In the end, these concerns were relieved when the Court upheld the ACA in a 6–3 vote.

However, the existential legal challenges to Obamacare did not end with Obama's presidency. In early 2018, Texas and nineteen other states sued the federal government on the basis that the individual mandate was unconstitutional because the 2017 Tax Cuts and Jobs Act had reduced the penalty for non-compliance with the mandate to zero dollars.[11] When the Trump administration effectively declined to defend the federal law, a second group of states stepped in to do so. Seventeen states, led by California, joined the legal opposition to the attack on the ACA, thus pitting states against states in this legal contest. In December 2020, a federal judge in Texas sided with the plaintiffs and said the whole ACA should be struck down as a consequence. Ken Paxton, the attorney general of Texas, quickly revived the dissenting rhetoric of many Republican leaders ten years earlier and declared that "today's ruling enjoining Obamacare halts an unconstitutional exertion of federal power over the American health care system."[12] The law stayed in place pending appeal and the case proceeded to the Supreme Court. In its decision, the Court avoided the merits of the argument and by 7–2 majority ruled that the plaintiffs did not have standing to bring the case.[13] Justice Alito penned a sharp dissent insisting that the whole law should have been struck down, but there was otherwise little protest from the wider conservative commentariat—a marked difference compared to the vehement responses to Chief Justice Roberts's decision to uphold the overall constitutionality of the ACA in 2012.

States have also remained a key source of struggle over health insurance since 2016. And, as *Obamacare Wars* suggests, the ACA's design has meant that these struggles vary significantly across the core components of the law. We first turn to the ACA's insurance exchanges. Even as public opinion on the ACA has improved, states' participation in this portion of the law has remained relatively constant. After more than a decade, thirty states have opted not to create their own state-based marketplaces, defaulting instead to the federally facilitated marketplace.[14] This continued pattern reflects the challenges we document in this book. Not only did partisanship hamper the development of state-based marketplaces, the preexisting policy legacies and a high level of institutional fragmentation have also weighed heavily against the creation of exchanges, even in some states where support for the ACA is strong.[15]

States' default to the federally facilitated marketplace has had significant policy consequences. On average, states that decided to implement their own marketplaces witness lower insurance premiums, fewer carrier exits, and more stable enrollment than states that chose to let the federal government do all the work.[16] At the same time, congressional intransigence in improving the ACA has allowed unintended and perverse dynamics to proliferate, even in state-based marketplaces. Arguably the most important example of this was the "subsidy cliff." Because of the ACA's means-tested structure that only provided subsidies for the purchase of insurance to individuals making less than $51,000 per year, middle-class people without insurance remained highly vulnerable to market dynamics. The only options for many individuals making just above the income cutoff were health plans that cost 20 percent of their annual income or more. Not only did this policy design prevent individuals from receiving affordable coverage, it also impeded states from adding their own subsidies. As one state-level policy advocate put it, the subsidy cliff served as a policy straitjacket "where the more you struggle the tighter it gets."[17] It was not until the passage of the American Rescue Plan Act—the Biden administration's first major legislative achievement—that Congress temporarily lifted the income cap on subsidies, which meant no American citizen would be required to pay more than 8.5 percent of their income on insurance. A little over a year later, as part of the Inflation Reduction Act, Congress extended this change until 2025.[18]

Since 2016, Medicaid expansion has become an increasingly dynamic arena for political struggle. This has hinged on preexisting policy legacies. As we note in the book, Medicaid waivers under Section 1115 of the Social Security Act were one way the Obama administration attempted to entice Republican governors to expand Medicaid. The Trump administration, by contrast, leveraged Section 1115 waivers to reverse coverage expansion by allowing states to require employment as a condition of Medicaid eligibility. Twenty-two states ultimately submitted applications for work requirements within Medicaid, thirteen of which were approved.[19] A barrage of lawsuits, combined with the election of Democratic governors in applicant states like Maine and Kentucky, halted the implementation of these waivers. Only one state, Arkansas, ever fully implemented such a waiver, resulting in coverage loss for 18,000 beneficiaries.[20] By 2019, the DC Circuit Court of Appeals held that these waivers violated the Medicaid statute.[21]

While the ACA's opponents attempted to use waivers to reduce insurance coverage, albeit unsuccessfully, supporters of the law used another institution, the ballot initiative, to expand it. Between 2017 and 2021, every state that successfully expanded Medicaid did so through a ballot initiative approved by voters. Ballot initiatives allow voters to engage in conflict expansion, transforming the issue of Medicaid expansion from a partisan fight among elected officials into a referendum on a benefit that is broadly popular even in Republican strongholds. Across the six states where Medicaid expansion was on the ballot, it received a higher share of support than the 2016 Democratic presidential candidate in all but eight counties.[22]

The ballot initiative, despite its promise as a mechanism for policy change, is (as of the writing of this preface) available in only three of the eleven states that have not yet expanded Medicaid. In the rest, expansion will hinge on engagement in Republican-dominated state legislatures where support for expansion has been frosty at best, even in places where major health-sector coalitions exist. If past is prologue, these efforts will also be shaped in significant ways by a highly racialized politics, something which the analysis in our book neglects. Even so, there is strong evidence to suggest that racial resentment has impeded the passage of Medicaid expansions, especially in Republican-governed states with large Black populations.[23]

The ACA's regulatory reforms, unlike the dynamic issues of insurance exchanges and Medicaid expansion, have demonstrated a certain amount of stability in recent years. Though the law's protections for individuals with preexisting conditions were not initially salient, the threat of repeal that followed Republicans' 2016 electoral victory helped enhance its visibility and public approval, despite the fact that other dimensions of the law remained controversial.[24] Hence, even as the Trump administration sought to undermine the ACA in other ways, it generally enforced existing consumer protections, even threatening to take over enforcement in states that attempted to skirt compliance.[25] On the other hand, the Trump administration did attempt to sabotage the ACA's regulatory reforms not through direct repeal but by reinterpreting statutory provisions in ways that undermined their effectiveness. One such attempt was relaxing prohibitions on the sale of cheap, low-quality coverage plans—a move many analysts feared would entice healthy customers out of the ACA's marketplaces, resulting in higher premiums and weaker consumer protections.[26] Additionally, the Trump administration suspended enforcement of regulations that ensured ACA marketplaces would have healthcare networks with adequate numbers and types of providers to serve enrollees.[27] In the end, these efforts yielded marginal increases in the number of uninsured people but did not produce anything like a reversion to the pre-ACA status quo.[28]

In the post-Obama era, the word "Obamacare" (first devised by Republican strategist Frank Luntz) ceased to play the role the ACA's opponents had intended. However tenacious, efforts to repeal and replace the law and even persistent attempts at sabotage have done little to jeopardize the long-term political stability of this major reform. At the same time, these efforts helped to keep the ACA's supporters fighting rearguard attacks, frustrating attempts to realize the vision of the law (to say nothing of expanding that vision). Most importantly, the ACA's fragmented structure has produced multiple political dynamics across various dimensions of the law. In fact, the turbulence that has defined policymaking in the years since *Obamacare Wars* was first published, including variations in policy legacies, institutional fragmentation, and public sentiments, has continued to shape the law's trajectory at the state level. However politically stable the law has been on the national scale, this fragmented structure has continued to produce significant disparities in coverage across the states.

Whatever the future of the ACA, or of health reform more generally, our book continues to provide clear lessons here for those who design and implement major reforms. In environments of intense political contestation, designing policy with weak legacies and fragmented institutional designs opens up vulnerabilities that are not easily addressed with traditional policy tools. Intergovernmental grants, consultation procedures, and regulatory clarity still matter, of course. Yet when intense political conflict persists after enactment, especially when implementation is decentralized, the task of political persuasion and coalition building remains. The avenues available to those seeking to persuade lawmakers and build coalitions certainly vary according to institutional arrangements. Back in South Dakota, the Republican governing political class remained opposed to any expansion of the state's Medicaid program, but advocates for change succeeded in getting an initiative for a constitutional amendment on the ballot for November 2022. Because it was successful, this initiative to join the ACA's Medicaid expansion should lead to at least 40,000 South Dakotans getting access to health coverage.[29] This was not how President Obama saw events unfolding when he signed the ACA into law, but no reform—and certainly not one as significant as the ACA—has ever been self-implementing.

Daniel Béland, Philip Rocco, and Alex Waddan
December 2022

NOTES

1. Daniel Bush, "Support for Medicaid expansion grows in South Dakota, one of the last red state holdouts," PBS News Hour, March 16, 2021, https://www.pbs.org/newshour/health/support-for-medicaid-expansion-grows-in-south-dakota-one-of-the-last-red-state-holdouts; Laura Santhanam, "South Dakota passed Medicaid expansion. What's next?" PBS News Hour, November 15, 2022, https://www.pbs.org/newshour/health/south-dakota-passed-medicaid-expansion-whats-next.

2. CDC/NCHS, National Health Interview Survey, reported in http://www.cdc.gov/nchs/health_policy/trends_hc_1968_2011.htm#table01 and https://www.cdc.gov/nchs/data/nhis/earlyrelease/Insur201808.pdf; "Health Insurance Coverage of Nonelderly 06–4 (CPS)," Kaiser Family Foundation, https://www.kff.org/other/state-indicator/health-insurance-coverage-of-nonelderly-06–4/?currentTimeframe=0&sortModel=%7B%22colId%22:%22Uninsured%22,%22sort%22:%22desc%22%7D.

3. Benjamin D. Sommers, "State Medicaid expansions and mortality, revisited: a cost-benefit analysis," *American Journal of Health Economics* 3 (3, 2017): 392–421.

4. Eric Patashnik, *Reforms at Risk: What Happens After Major Policy Changes are Enacted* (Princeton, NJ: Princeton University Press, 2008).

5. Lilliana Mason, *Uncivil Agreement: How Politics Became Our Identity* (Princeton, NJ: Princeton University Press, 2018).

6. This analysis draws in part on Daniel Béland, Philip Rocco, and Alex Waddan, "The Affordable Care Act in the States: Fragmented Politics, Unstable Policy," *Journal of Health Politics, Policy and Law* 45, no. 4 (2020): 647–660.

7. Daniel Béland, Philip Rocco, and Alex Waddan, "Obamacare in the Trump Era: Where are we Now, and Where are we Going?," *The Political Quarterly* 89, no. 4 (2018): 687–694; Philip Rocco and Simon F. Haeder, "How intense policy demanders shape postreform politics: Evidence from the Affordable Care Act," *Journal of Health Politics, Policy and Law* 43, no. 2 (2018): 271–304.

8. Suzanne Mettler, Lawrence R. Jacobs, and Ling Zhu, "Policy Threat, Partisanship, and the Case of the Affordable Care Act," *American Political Science Review* (2022).

9. Linda J. Blumberg, Matthew Buettgens, and John Holahan, "The Implications of a Supreme Court Finding for the Plaintiff in King vs. Burwell: 8.2 Million More Uninsured and 35% Higher Premiums," Robert Wood Johnson Foundation and the Urban Institute, January 2015, https://www.urban.org/sites/default/files/publication/49246/2000062-The-Implications-King-vs-Burwell.pdf.

10. Nicholas Bagley, David K. Jones, and Timothy S. Jost, "Predicting the Fallout from *King v. Burwell*: Exchanges and the ACA," *New England Journal of Medicine* 372 (2015): 101–104.

11. Congressional Budget Office, H.R. 1, The Tax Cuts and Jobs Act, Cost Estimate, November 13, 2017, https://www.cbo.gov/publication/53312, accessed 1 September 2022.

12. Abby Goodnough and Robert Pear, "Texas Judge Strikes Down Obama's Affordable Care Act as Unconstitutional," *New York Times,* December 14, 2018, https://www.nytimes.com/2018/12/14/health/obamacare-unconstitutional-texas-judge.html.

13. Nicholas Bagley J.D. "*California v. Texas*—Ending the Campaign to Undo the ACA in the Courts," *New England Journal of Medicine* 385 (2021): 673–675.

14. Kaiser Family Foundation, "State Health Insurance Marketplace Types, 2022," https://www.kff.org/health-reform/state-indicator/state-health-insurance-marketplace-types/?current Timeframe=0&sortModel=%7B%22colId%22:%22Location%22,%22sort%22:%22asc%22%7D, accessed 1 September 2022.

15. David K. Jones, Sarah H. Gordon, and Nicole Huberfeld, "Have the ACA's Exchanges Succeeded? It's Complicated," *Journal of Health Politics, Policy, and Law* 45, no. 4 (2020): 661–676.

16. Jane M. Zhu, Daniel Polsky, and Yuehan Zhang, "State-Based Marketplaces Outperform Federally-Facilitated Marketplaces," Leonard Davis Institute of Health Economics, Issue Brief, March 2018, https://ldi.upenn.edu/wp-content/uploads/archive/pdf/LDI%20Issue%20Brief%20 2018%20No.%201_6.pdf.

17. Jon Walker, "The Almost Big F*cking Deal in the COVID Relief Bill," *The American Prospect,* March 9, 2021, https://prospect.org/health/covid-relief-bill-health-insurance-subsidy-cliff/.

18. Cynthia Cox, Krutika Amin, and Jared Ortalitza, "Five Things to Know about the Renewal of Extra Affordable Care Act Subsidies in the Inflation Reduction Act," Kaiser Family Foundation, August 11, 2022, https://www.kff.org/policy-watch/five-things-to-know-about-re newal-of-extra-affordable-care-act-subsidies-in-inflation-reduction-act/.

19. "Medicaid Waiver Tracker: Approved and Pending Section 1115 Waivers by State," Kaiser Family Foundation, August 19, 2022, https://www.kff.org/report-section/section-1115-waiver -tracker-work-requirements/.

20. Benjamin D. Sommers, Anna L. Goldman, Robert J. Blendon, E. John Orav, and Arnold M. Epstein, "Medicaid work requirements—results from the first year in Arkansas," *New England Journal of Medicine* 381, no. 11 (2019): 1073–1082.

21. *Gresham v. Azar,* No. 195-094 (D.C. Cir. 2020).

22. Philip Rocco, "Direct Democracy and the Fate of Medicaid Expansion," *JAMA Health Forum,* August 21, 2020.

23. Jamila Michener, "Race Politics and the Affordable Care Act," *Journal of Health Politics, Policy, and Law* 45, no. 4 (2020): 547–566; Colleen M. Grogan and Sunggeun Park, "The Racial Divide in State Medicaid Expansions," *Journal of Health Politics, Policy and Law* 42, no. 3 (2017): 539–572.

24. Mark A. Peterson, "Reversing Course on Obamacare: Why Not Another Medicare Catastrophic?," *Journal of Health Politics, Policy, and Law* 43, no. 4 (2018): 605–650.

25. Robert Pear, "Trump Administration Blocks Idaho's Plan to Circumvent Health Law," *New York Times,* March 8, 2018.

26. James M. Brasfield, *The Affordable Care Act: At the Nexus of Policy and Politics* (Boulder, CO: Lynne Rienner, 2022), 141–167.

27. Justin Giovanelli, "Ensuring the Adequacy of ACA Marketplace Plan Networks," Commonwealth Fund blog, February 15, 2022, https://www.commonwealthfund.org/blog/2022/ensur ing-adequacy-aca-marketplace-plan-networks.

28. Of course, had the arguments in *Texas v. United States* prevailed at the Supreme Court, state regulatory policies would have been thrown into chaos. While many states came into compliance with the ACA without extensive legislative or gubernatorial involvement, fewer than half the states enacted legislation specifically enshrining community ratings, guaranteed issue, and bans on preexisting condition exclusion. Corlette and Curran 2019.

29. Lee Strubinger, "Health care advocates join to back one Medicaid expansion ballot question, instead of two," South Dakota Public Broadcasting, July 11, 2022, https://listen.sdpb.org /politics/20220-71-1/health-care-advocates-join-to-back-one-medicaid-expansion-ballot-ques tion-instead-of-two.

PREFACE TO THE FIRST EDITION

The Patient Protection and Affordable Care Act (ACA) is by far the most crucial health care reform enacted in the United States since the adoption of Medicare and Medicaid in 1965. One of the most striking things about the ACA is the intense political battle that has surrounded this reform, both before and since President Barack Obama signed it into law in March 2010. In the United States, health care reform is very much an unfinished fight, and our book is devoted to the politics surrounding the implementation of the ACA in the four years following its enactment.

This project began shortly after Daniel Béland and Phil Rocco met for the first time, during the 2013 meeting of the American Political Science Association, and realized we were both captivated by the ongoing politics of health care reform and that some collaborative work on the topic should take place. Through a flurry of e-mails exchanged in the days following that Chicago meeting, Alex Waddan became involved in a conversation that would soon convince the three of us we should write a book on the topic. The project moved rapidly because we each had already conducted extensive research on the ACA.

From the beginning of our conversation, it became clear we wanted to focus on federalism and the politics of implementing the ACA in the fifty states. Although politics at the national level and legal challenges to the constitutionality of the ACA are fascinating and crucial in shaping the implementation of the ACA, we wanted to study the politics of health care reform in the states to account for diverging patterns of consent and dissent in implementing the ACA. As we began working on this book, we decided to focus on three major policy streams central to the effective application of the ACA: the creation of health insurance exchanges offering affordable insurance packages with government subsidies to low-income Americans not eligible for Medicaid, the expansion of Medicaid to cover those with incomes up to 138 percent of the federal poverty level, and regulatory reform designed to limit insurance premium increases and compel insurers to spend most of their revenues on medical care. In each of these areas state-level actors were required to act to make the law work effectively. As we show through this book, the law's extended and highly contentious implementation process caused those state actors to behave in ways that varied dramatically across the distinctive policy streams of the reform.

Conducting interviews and looking at the evidence available from both quantitative data and the set of case studies we examined, we noticed that these variations resulted from more than the states' political inclinations or idiosyncratic features of the state reform contexts. Each of these three streams operated according to a different political logic. Although we recognized that what happens in one of the ACA reform streams could affect the situation in another stream, it proved clear to us that patterns of consent and cooperation characterized regulatory reform, a situation that contrasted with Medicaid reform and, especially, health insurance exchanges, which witnessed much more dissent and much less cooperation. Especially striking to us was the fact that these political differences across reform streams are sometimes present even within the same state. By emphasizing the diversity of the politics of the ACA in the states, our book contributes to knowledge about how and why such consequential health care reform is unevenly implemented across the fifty states.

We chose to limit our study to the first four years of the ACA's implementation. Although we knew debates about the ACA would be ongoing, and interpretations of its history would continue to evolve as new evidence came to light, we believed that, in light of prior scholarship, four years set an important first benchmark for how the federal system responded to major reforms. Moreover, although the ACA's politics and policy may change in the future, its uneven implementation thus far has had direct and sometimes dramatic consequences on the ground for the well-being and economic security of millions of Americans. Although our book focuses on federalism and state politics, we understand that the key political decisions under investigation made in the fifty state capitals can have a profound and deeply felt impact on large segments of the population, which is why this politics matters so much and deserves close, comparative examination. We hope our book can help the reader better grasp why state officials made the decisions they did and why the implementation of the ACA is taking the sinuous path it is across the fifty states, in what remains a geographically fragmented health care system. As we suggest, studying state politics in a comparative perspective is a most insightful way to grasp the evolution of this system.

A number of great people directly assisted us in preparing this book. First, we thank Rachel Hatcher, Dylan Clark, Bo Kovitz, and Ishmael Wireko for their editorial and research assistance. Second, we are grateful to Weiping Zeng and the Spatial Initiative at the University of Saskatchewan for helping us prepare the maps featured in this book. Third, we thank the people who agreed to be interviewed as part of this project for their insight. Fourth, the reviewers provided most helpful feedback on our manuscript, which was significantly improved as a consequence. Thank you to them for taking the time to read our manuscript so carefully, and for offering both detailed and constructive comments. Fifth, at the University Press of Kansas, Fred Woodward and Chuck Myers provided admirable guidance and support, from the initial stage of this project to the publication process. We warmly thank them and the rest of the Kansas team, whose hard work has helped to launch numerous landmark studies in the field of American politics. Finally, Daniel Béland acknowledges support from the Canada Research Chairs Program, and Phil Rocco acknowledges the Institute of Governmental Studies, which has supported his research at the University of California, Berkeley.

Permission to use material from the following publication is gratefully acknowledged: Daniel Béland, Philip Rocco, and Alex Waddan, "Implementing Health Care Reform in the United States: Intergovernmental Politics and the Dilemmas of Institutional Design," *Health Policy* 116, no. 1 (2014): 51–60.

Introduction

The battle over health care reform in the United States did not, as its supporters hoped, end with the adoption of the Patient Protection and Affordable Care Act (ACA) in March 2010. The very day President Barack Obama signed the ACA into law, a number of states made it clear they would challenge the law in court. As the *Washington Post* reported, "Not five minutes after President Obama signed health-care legislation into law . . . , top staff members for Virginia Attorney General Ken Cuccinelli II made their way out of his office, court papers in hand and TV cameras in pursuit, and headed to Richmond's federal courthouse to sue to stop the measure."[1] As the initial flurry of state lawsuits against the ACA suggested, health care reform opponents decided to strike back hard and fast, using powerful language to express their hostility toward the federal health care reform. Speaking at a conference held by the American Enterprise Institute in December 2010, conservative legal scholar Michael Greve issued a challenge to his colleagues in these blunt terms:

> This bastard [the ACA] has to be killed as a matter of political hygiene. I do not care how this is done, whether it's dismembered, whether we drive a stake through its heart, whether we tar and feather it and drive it out of town, whether we strangle it. I don't care who does it, whether it's some court some place [*sic*], or the United States Congress. Any which way, any dollar spent on that goal is worth spending, any brief filed toward that end is worth filing, any speech or panel contribution toward that end is of service to the United States.[2]

Greve's speech was only the beginning of a much larger attack on health care reform that, even four years after the ACA became the law of the land, has persisted. This is why, on April 1, 2014, just after the law's first open-enrollment period, President Obama felt the need to publicly defend the ACA, as he had on numerous occasions since he signed the legislation. At the core of this 2014 speech was his claim that the "Affordable Care Act is here to stay" and his statement that "those who have based their entire political agenda on repealing" the ACA should explain to people who already benefit from it why they want to repeal it. Importantly, he also claimed Americans "can stop refighting old political battles that keep us gridlocked," a statement that points to lasting political dissent over the ACA, both at the national and at the state levels.[3]

An enduringly controversial law, the ACA aims to gradually reduce the number of people in the United States who are uninsured, which stood at around 50 million in 2010, and to control spiraling costs associated with providing health care here. To do so, the government regulates the private insurance sector by scrutinizing prices and mandating broader access to coverage, creating health insurance exchanges to help individuals and small businesses purchase insurance, and making provisions for a large expansion of Medicaid, the state-run health insurance program for the poor. Yet the ACA's passage alone did not guarantee the achievement of these goals. The most important health care reform since the adoption of Medicaid and Medicare in 1965, the ACA is a complex and multifaceted piece of legislation, with rollout set to take place gradually over nearly a decade, through 2019. Because of this extended time frame, the complexity of the legislation, the central role of states in its implementation, and the enduring political opposition discussed above, the enactment of the ACA was not the end but rather the beginning of a new chapter in the fight over health care reform.

In this context, opponents such as the National Federation of Independent Business (NFIB), insurance companies, Tea Party supporters, and conservative activists quickly mobilized across the institutional terrain of the US government—in the courts, at notice-and-comment sessions in federal agencies, in state capitals, and in the public sphere—to contest the reform before it could take root. Each of these constituencies had different reasons to oppose the ACA. For instance, the NFIB took issue with requirements for employers, insurance companies disliked key aspects of regulatory reform, and Tea Party and conservative activists rejected the entire package. Despite their differences of opinion, opponents were not deterred by the enactment of the ACA. Instead, they organized across the country to stall or, at least complicate and undermine, its implementation.[4] The importance of this postenactment opposition became especially clear in fall 2013, when the obstacles put in place contributed in part to a problematic rollout of key aspects of the law, such as the proposed Medicaid expansion and the creation of health insurance exchanges. Here it is crucial to understand that opponents have mobilized politically in different ways with different levels of success, depending on the issue at hand. For instance, by April 2014, although half of the states agreed to expand Medicaid, barely a third of them decided to set up their own health insurance exchanges.

In this book, we argue that opponents of the ACA have used the US federal system to continue the fight over health care reform in ways that vary across the major components of the law. The ACA's institutional structure enables this contestation. To ensure that the bill would be perceived as a moderate reform, seemingly radical alternatives favored by the left of the Democratic Party, such as a single-payer system, were never seriously contemplated. Even more expansive versions of provisions on the table, such as a single, federally run health insurance exchange, were excised from the final form of the legislation.[5] As Eric Patashnik and Julian Zelizer have noted, the ACA did not restructure political institutions or health insurance markets in a way that would have destroyed opposition to health care reform.[6] Thus, the law did not centralize health care arrangements in the manner championed by the many liberal advocates of reform. It did not establish anything resembling "Medicare for all," which would have left the federal government as the dominant player in the organization of health care. In fact, rather than simplifying the already extraordinarily complex system, the ACA depended on integrating more layers into the existing policy fabric. Most importantly, the ACA dispersed governing authority to a patchwork of state governors, legislatures, and regulatory agencies with which the Department of Health and Human Services (HHS) had to collaborate.[7] As our book shows, these state-level policy makers were often simply unwilling to cooperate in the law's application. Hence the ACA's complex design and delegation of implementation created a window of opportunity for its opponents at the state level to shape, and in some cases obstruct, implementation. In 2010, parties and groups opposed to the ACA poured their energies into state electoral contests, contributing to significant Republican gains and leaving a state implementation context divided along partisan lines.

Importantly, however, elected officials at the state level did not have equal opportunities to obstruct *all* of the relevant provisions of the ACA. The ACA is not a coherent reform; rather, it is a bundle of policy changes with their own political logic and institutional structures. Most importantly, each stream of reform within the ACA—health insurance exchanges, Medicaid expansion, and regulatory reform—interacts with the federal system in a different way because each is associated with unique policy legacies, institutional settings, and public sentiments.[8] These variations, we argue, made some reform streams more vulnerable to state-level contestation than others did. Our book compares and contrasts how state elected officials behaved within three of these reform streams, all of which are major components of the ACA that depend crucially on the involvement of state governments. In particular, we focus on the development of health insurance exchanges (also known as health insurance marketplaces), the expansion of Medicaid, and the introduction of new health insurance regulations.

Through a detailed analysis of the policy legacies, institutional settings, and public sentiments that characterize each of these reform streams, we explain why the state-level politics of ACA implementation has varied across the exchanges, Medicaid, and regulatory reforms. After formulating a coherent analytical framework to study the politics of implementation in an intergovernmental context, we compare and contrast state-level debates and actions in relation to these three streams from the signing of the ACA in late March 2010 to the end of the first open-enrollment period in late March 2014.

Our comparative analysis reveals important divergences in the politics of the three reform streams under consideration. The implementation of reform in each of the different streams under consideration did not take place in a sealed-off policy silo, completely detached from developments elsewhere. The wider political fight over the ACA's legitimacy clearly affected the decision making of state policy makers and other stakeholders across all the streams, be they emboldened in their resistance to the law or encouraged to collaborate with the federal authorities. Yet, as we show, actors were constrained or enabled by the implementation dynamics in each stream. Different institutional configurations and varied incentives framed how those involved viewed the costs and benefits of cooperation or opposition to building exchanges, expanding Medicaid, or enforcing regulatory reform. Out of these streams, the politics of health insurance exchanges has triggered the most dissent and intergovernmental conflict. In sharp contrast, the implementation of regulatory policy has typically taken the form of bargaining among policy elites over the details of reform, resulting in the emergence of wide consent among states to implement weaker reforms. Furthermore, we suggest that Medicaid expansion is a more controversial issue than regulatory reform for the states. Yet this reform stream brings a greater level of state participation than do health insurance exchanges, which have the strongest level of conflict over implementation, largely because of a robust legacy of state-federal collaboration on Medicaid. Nevertheless, the refusal of states to participate in Medicaid expansion has much more direct consequences on citizens than the refusal of states to set up their own health insurance exchanges, where the federal government can simply act on its own. This option is not available in the Medicaid reform stream, in which state action is required to implement expansion for potentially newly eligible individuals. Thus, in terms of a clear contrast between recurrent dissent (Medicaid, exchanges) and negotiated consent (regulatory reform), the politics of ACA implementation varies greatly from one reform stream to another, a situation our comparative analysis both describes and explains.

Beyond widening our understanding of the politics of ACA implementation, our book draws broader lessons for the analysis of federalism and intergovernmental politics in the United States. First, our analysis points to the fact that the federal system is not one unified, homogenous constitutional battlefield but rather many distinct policy battlefields, each characterized by its own political logic. Factors such as policy legacies, institutional configurations, and public sentiments all shape politics in the federal system. Second, the very nature of this political logic tends to direct the tactics of state actors during policy implementation. Third, these tactics are not homogeneous but diverse in nature because they involve consent, dissent, or a combination of both. Finally, in the politics of intergovernmental policy implementation, different kinds of contestation feature different actors, audiences, and probabilities of victory for opponents of the reform at stake.

THE ENDURING CHALLENGE OF HEALTH CARE REFORM

Grasping the politics of ACA implementation requires an understanding of the multifaceted problems the US health care system faced before the reform was even conceived. In reality, the problems President Obama and his allies set out to remedy had long been in the making. When Governor Bill Clinton was campaigning for the presidency in 1992, he denounced a system that left "60 million Americans without adequate health insurance and bankrupts our families, our businesses, and our federal budget."[9] In 1993, 39.7 million Americans, amounting to 15.3 percent of the population, were uninsured;[10] yet the United States, in devoting 13 percent of its gross domestic product (GDP) to health care, spent more on health care than any other industrialized nation.[11] Clinton's failure to correct these issues led some commentators to conclude that the institutional fragmentation of the US government prevented the enactment of a comprehensive reform package in Washington, DC.[12] Yet, fifteen years later, during the 2008 campaign and at the beginning of the Obama presidency, the problems of access and cost had worsened enough that Democrats felt that health care reform had once again become too pressing an issue to ignore.

After the legislative debacle of the Health Security Act, the Clinton administration managed to push through some incremental health reforms that helped improve access to care for a few groups. The Health Insurance Portability and Accountability Act (HIPAA), enacted in 1996, made it easier for workers, particularly those with preexisting medical conditions, to keep their insurance if they changed jobs.[13] Additionally, the State Children's Health Insurance Program (SCHIP, now known as CHIP) expanded access to health care for children living in households with incomes up to 200 percent of the federal poverty level but whose parent or guardian could not afford to purchase private insurance.[14] This program, which allocated $24 billion over five years through block grants to the states, represented the "nation's largest publicly funded health insurance expansion" since the creation of Medicare and Medicaid in the mid-1960s.[15] Despite the uneven implementation of SCHIP, by 2006 an estimated 6.7 million children were benefiting from the program.[16] Yet, the number of uninsured Americans remained constant. In the wake of the passage of HIPAA, President Clinton claimed that the law represented a "long step toward the kind of health care our nation needs."[17] However, in reality, whatever the merits were of the measures passed in the 1990s, 14.9 percent of Americans were still uninsured in 2008.[18] In addition, many millions more were underinsured and faced the possibility of huge, potentially unaffordable costs if they needed health care.[19]

In addition to no significant reduction in the proportion of Americans lacking insurance in the years since President Clinton's reform initiative, the intervening years had brought a continuing escalation of health care costs. By 2008, health care costs had risen to 16 percent of the GDP, reinforcing the country's status as the biggest health care spender in the world. In terms of universal coverage, France spent 11.2 percent, Germany 10.5 percent, and the United Kingdom 8.7 percent of their respective GDPs on health care.[20] In January 2010, as the ACA was still in the legislative process, the Congressional Budget Office (CBO) warned, "The biggest single threat to budgetary stability is the growth of federal spending on health care—pushed up both by increases in the number of beneficiaries of Medicare and Medicaid (because of the aging of the population) and by growth in spending per beneficiary that outstrips growth in per capita GDP."[21] Furthermore, state governments were becoming increasingly concerned over how to sustain their contribution to Medicaid, with state officials forced into uncomfortable choices between spending on health care coverage for low-income constituents and other crucial expenditures.[22] In addition, although they typically passed on some of the increase in health care costs to consumers and workers, employers who offered insurance to their employees became increasingly worried about the rise in such costs.[23] For example, by the mid-2000s, Starbucks was spending more money on health insurance for its employees than it was spending on coffee beans.[24] These pressures meant that the long-term viability of the employer-based model of insurance had to be questioned.[25] In 2000, 65.1 percent of Americans enjoyed employment-based insurance, but this number had diminished to 56.1 percent in 2009.[26]

These aggregate numbers about the uninsured and costs of care were widely cited in the public domain, fueling pressure on the federal government to take action.[27] Importantly, however, the number of uninsured Americans did not represent a balanced cross section of society. Unsurprisingly, the disparities within the US economy are reflected in the demographic composition of the uninsured; focusing only on the overall number of people uninsured tends to overlook significant discrepancies in access to health insurance by their race and ethnicity. For example, in a 2002 report commissioned by Congress, the Institute of Medicine commented:

> There are wide differences between racial and ethnic groups in access to health care and the availability of health insurance. Minorities, especially Hispanic and African-American families, are less likely than whites to have private health insurance. Or if they have insurance, minorities are more likely than whites to be enrolled in health plans that place tight limits on the types of services that patients may receive. Also, the best quality health care services and providers are not always found in minority communities.[28]

Six years later, when President Obama was elected in 2008, these inequities remained acute. The rate of uninsured among white, non-Hispanic Americans was 10.8 percent. Of African Americans, 19.1 percent were uninsured, whereas for people of Hispanic origin that number was higher still, at an astonishing 30.7 percent.[29] A key aspect of these discrepancies was that African Americans and Hispanics were significantly less likely to have access to employer-related insurance. In 2008, 65 percent of white Americans had some kind of employer-related insurance, but for African Americans and Hispanics the numbers were 48.8 percent and 41 percent, respectively.[30]

These numbers matter in part because of their social significance but also because of their potential impact on how political actors might construe the likely "winners" of health care reform.[31] For all the worries about the uninsured, most Americans did have insurance, and in designing any reform it was important for reformers not to appear to be threatening existing insurance coverage. One cross-national survey of people's opinions of health care arrangements in their own countries is especially revealing about contradictory tensions policy makers in the United States faced when crafting a reform package. US respondents to the survey were the most likely to say their country's health care system needed major surgery, but they were also the most likely to express confidence in the quality of treatment available: "Compared with the other 10 countries, the U.S. had the highest percentage of respondents who reported being very confident they would receive effective treatment (34.7%) and also the highest percentage saying they were not at all confident they would (9.2%)."[32]

This combination of factors made the task of devising comprehensive change highly problematic. This was the case because reformers needed to prove they could simultaneously control health care costs and expand access to health insurance for millions of Americans without appearing to threaten the arrangements of those already satisfied with their insurance. Furthermore, within the political arena, as President Clinton had discovered, coming up with a blueprint for reform was the easy part when compared with the task of getting Congress to make a serious effort at legislating it.

When the time came to design health care reform at the outset of Obama's presidency, however, significant variation existed in the policy legacies of insurance exchanges, Medicaid, and regulatory reform. These policy legacies had an impact on the content of the final legislation adopted in March 2010. First, concerning health insurance exchanges, ideas such as individual mandates and purchasing pools had long been popular within policy circles, including conservative ones. Some of these ideas influenced the 2006 Massachusetts health insurance reform, sometimes known as "Romneycare," a platform viewed as bipartisan because both Democratic state legislators and Republican governor Mitt Romney ended up supporting it.[33] Nevertheless, virtually no states had followed the lead of Massachusetts in making these ideas into concrete policy reforms. Second, since the 1980s,

Medicaid had expanded significantly as a program, and, in the year preceding the enactment of the ACA, a number of reform advocates had pushed for expanding it further to reduce the number of uninsured among low-income Americans.[34] Finally, when it came to regulatory reform, both the states and the federal government had already begun experimenting with rate regulation and the medical loss ratio (MLR), which involves submitting "data on the proportion of premium revenues spent on clinical services and quality improvement."[35] Thus, the three reform components on which we focus—health insurance exchanges, Medicaid expansion, and regulatory reform—already enjoyed some level of elite support before the enactment process for the ACA even began. Nevertheless, as the reform effort took shape in 2009, strengthened GOP opposition would undermine this consensus and lead to a much more contentious process of enactment and implementation.

During the prolonged and highly divisive political process that led to the enactment of the ACA, what was at stake became increasingly clear as both controlling costs and extending coverage in a world of complex policy legacies, powerful vested interests, and GOP opposition proved a difficult task. If anything, President Obama's choice to allow Congress to prepare a detailed policy blueprint instead of providing one himself, as President Clinton had done fifteen years earlier, slowed down an already slow-moving enactment process. This situation explains why the surprise election of Republican Scott Brown to the Senate in January 2010 was so disruptive, because Democrats lost their supermajority of sixty seats before the final compromise between the House and the Senate bills. In the end, in the absence of Republican support for the legislation, this turn of events forced Democrats to adopt the Senate version of the legislation, which featured a more decentralized approach to health care reform than the House version. In particular, in terms of the health insurance exchanges, Congress did not adopt the purely national approach featured in the House bill but rather a system in which states could set up their own exchanges. This choice paved the way for significant policy disparities and inadvertently created a political window of opportunity for opponents of the ACA within the states to use their power over the creation of state-operated exchanges to express their discontent toward the federal legislation as a whole.

HOW POLICY LEGACIES, INSTITUTIONAL FRAGMENTATION, AND PUBLIC SENTIMENTS SHAPE POSTREFORM POLITICS

Because of the ACA's decentralized design, state-level electoral victories by Republicans in 2010 provided the leverage opponents needed to refight the battle over health care reform. Yet in contrast to existing scholarship on the politics of ACA implementation, we show evidence of wide variation in opponents' opportunities to challenge individual elements of health care reform. Although we agree with existing scholarship that partisanship and political polarization are driving forces of state governments' reaction to the ACA, our comparative analysis of intergovernmental politics reveals major differences in how opponents of the ACA responded to exchanges, Medicaid, and regulatory reforms. We argue that these variations are the result of three important factors: *policy legacies, the level of institutional fragmentation,* and *public sentiments.*

First, *policy legacies* consist of preexisting institutions and intergovernmental relationships that predate the passage of the ACA. Strong policy legacies act as a buttress against state-level opposition by raising the bar opponents must clear to stall reform. For instance, if a federal policy builds on popular reforms already undertaken at the state level, it may be difficult for opponents to build a coalition to reverse a "tide" of reform many years in the making. By contrast, weak policy legacies allow opponents of reform to leverage uncertainty about policy outcomes to sew doubt about embracing a new reform.

Policy legacies vary greatly across our three reform streams. For instance, whereas Medicaid is a well-established program associated with a long history of federal-state interactions, health insurance exchanges are a new policy instrument. The policy terrain of health insurance exchanges is both recent and undeveloped. Prior to the ACA, only Massachusetts had a working health insurance exchange. As for the policy legacies relevant to regulatory reform, states had more variable policy frameworks than in the Medicaid program in existence in most states since the late 1960s. Nevertheless, unlike in the case of the exchanges, most states had basic regulatory frameworks that aided in implementation.

A second focus in our analysis is *institutional fragmentation,* the extent to which a policy divides decision-making authority among multiple actors. Institutional fragmentation also varies considerably across our three cases. On the one hand, the most fragmented of these reform streams is health insurance exchanges. Health insurance exchanges, unlike Medicaid reform, featured weak fiscal incentives for states to participate and, unlike the lower profile of regulatory reform, necessitated highly visible state legislation to establish exchanges. On the other hand, regulatory reform is the most integrated and the least fragmented reform stream under consideration, in part because federal bodies have a stronger coercive capacity and because preexisting regulatory frameworks allowed state insurance departments to implement the reforms without additional action by state legislatures. We argue that institutional fragmentation empowers opponents of reform by allowing them to use institutional veto points to their advantage. If states must go to greater lengths to participate in federal reforms, and especially if they lack adequate incentives to do so, opponents may be able to fight back without much energy at all.

Finally, there are clear variations in *public sentiments*—defined as the public sa-lience of, and support for, a policy—across our three reform streams. For instance, regulatory reform has a very low public profile, whereas both Medicaid and health insurance exchanges are widely debated in the media and the political arena, thus making them highly visible to a divided public. As we show, high salience and mixed public support exacerbate political conflict over Medicaid and health insur-ance exchanges. By contrast, low salience in the regulatory reform stream fosters a politics of negotiated consent dominated by behind-the-scenes agreements be-tween state and federal officials.

These three types of contextual differences shape the political opportunities for dissent and consent in the politics of ACA implementation across the three reform streams we investigate. First, health insurance exchanges have faced high-profile but mixed public sentiments as well as the lowest level of consent and coopera-tion because of limited policy legacies in the states combined with institutionally fragmented reform that gives states the option to refuse to establish exchanges. In addition, many states simply refuse to create their own exchanges as a way of ex-pressing their opposition to the ACA. At the outset, opponents of the ACA in many states saw few downsides to this strategy. Although refusing to create exchanges would allow them to keep the debate about the ACA alive, they would suffer little blame for noncooperation, especially because the federal government would be-come responsible for establishing exchanges and providing premium tax credits to consumers in these states.[36] In fact, the failure of states to cooperate became the basis for a lengthy fight in federal courts in *King v. Burwell* (2015).

Second, Medicaid remains an intermediary case with its high public profile, making it more likely than regulatory reform to trigger heated political debates. However, Medicaid's well-established policy legacies and greater federal fiscal in-centives tend to somewhat mitigate conflict and generate a greater level of state consent, at least if measured in terms of the number of states that expanded their Medicaid programs compared with the number of states that established their own exchanges. Finally, in regulatory reform we observe negotiated consent rather than the politics of dissent. Opponents of these reforms found it more challeng-ing to engage in dissent because of deeper state policy legacies and an integrated institutional design combined with a low public profile that allows civil servants and other actors to bargain behind closed doors.

The divergent patterns of politics in the three streams we examine have sig-nificant policy consequences. For instance, although the existence of a federal "fallback" insurance exchange allowed citizens to purchase coverage regardless of states' cooperation, state dissent kept political conflict over the ACA alive and en-abled challenges to the ACA in federal courts, and ultimately the Supreme Court, regarding the applicability of premium-assistance tax credits in states that did not develop their own exchanges. Without these tax credits, enrollments in health care plans were projected to decline from 9.6 to 4.1 million, a decrease of 70 percent, and average premiums were projected to rise by 47 percent.[37] In June 2015, however, in a much-anticipated decision, the Supreme Court ruled that the law "authorized federal tax credits for eligible Americans living not only in states with their own exchanges but also in the 34 states with federal marketplaces."[38] However, state dissents on Medicaid pushed nearly 4 million poor, uninsured adults into a "coverage gap" because their income was too high to qualify them for current Medicaid benefits but below the lower limit for premium tax credits in the insurance marketplace.[39] Furthermore, states refusing to expand their Medicaid programs included Florida, where 1,253,000 people would potentially have become eligible for the program under the terms of the ACA; Texas with 1,186,000; and Georgia with 682,000. In contrast, in California, the decision to expand meant that more than 2.1 million people became newly eligible to register for Medicaid coverage.[40] Conversely, although states obviously varied in their approaches to enforcing the ACA's regulatory reforms, all but five states comply with the law, which means citizens can hold the vast majority of state governments accountable for consumer protection.[41]

In order to support our comparative claims, our methodological approach features a detailed analysis of policy legacies, institutional settings, and public sentiments across our three reform streams. Each of the three factors under consideration requires us to examine different sources of data, from court rulings, legislative texts, and media sources to interviews with policy makers and health care experts to public opinion data and academic studies. Gathering data on individual reform streams is not the end in itself because our goal is purely to grasp the political logic of ACA implementation in states as it varies *among* our three reform streams. Although our conclusions rely predominantly on qualitative case comparisons between reform streams, we also leverage descriptive quantitative data analysis for each individual stream to reveal broad patterns in the politics of implementation across all fifty states.

OVERVIEW

This book comprises five main chapters. The first chapter reviews and draws on the literature of federalism and intergovernmental relations to formulate the book's analytical framework, centered on the role of policy legacies, institutional settings, and public sentiments. The second chapter sets the scene for the politics of ACA implementation, describing how the institutional design of the reform created opportunities for its opponents to strike back at the state level and detailing how the 2010 elections made state elected officials potential veto players for the reform. Our assessment of the ACA's political context is followed by three chapters that apply our analytical framework to the politics of health insurance exchanges, Medicaid, and regulatory reform, respectively. These chapters illustrate the complex ways in which policy legacies, institutional settings, and public sentiments interacted in each of the three reform streams, framing how state policy makers perceived the incentives, opportunities, and threats contained in the ACA and how they reacted to those perceptions. As we show, these factors could push and pull in different directions, producing a variety of results across the states. The chapters on exchanges and Medicaid include case studies of events in selected states that provide insight into the reasoning that guided policy makers and help explain the logic behind what might seem like some counterintuitive developments in terms of whether states established their own insurance exchanges or expanded their Medicaid programs. The chapter on regulatory reform features only brief case studies but concentrates on early-stage negotiations and investigates how stakeholders negotiated their resistance, compromise, or cooperation with the requirements of the ACA. The book finishes with a short conclusion that directly compares and contrasts our three reform streams to further assess our claims about consent and dissent in the intergovernmental politics of ACA implementation.

1. Postreform Politics in the US Federal System: Patterns of Consent and Dissent

Four years after the passage of the Patient Protection and Affordable Care Act (ACA), "Repeal Obamacare" remained a Republican applause line. As the law's period for enrollment in insurance plans came to a close, governor and presidential hopeful Bobby Jindal (R-LA) put forward the "Freedom and Empowerment Plan," a twenty-four-page proposal filled with policy-driven arguments and citations from reputable studies.[1] His was one in a series of Republican plans to repeal the law and replace it with federal legislation that, among other things, would create private health savings accounts and give states flexibility to experiment with privatized health options for the low-income uninsured. To accomplish his plan, Jindal argued that state governments had to engage in *dissent*—in this case, formally refusing to participate in implementing major reform. As the governor put it, "Hopefully, states will rewrite their laws to eradicate Obamacare from their statute books."[2]

Jindal's suggestion drew on real-life examples because state declarations of opposition to the ACA's health insurance exchange provisions represented a central way in which Republican opponents of the ACA have engaged in what Eric Patashnik calls "postreform politics."[3] In hoping that governors and state legislatures would practice dissent, however, Jindal was also ignoring a crucial reality. Even in states where opposition to the ACA was strong, opponents also took another less visible approach to postreform politics: *negotiating their consent* to the ACA with federal officials. Whether during informal meetings between federal and state personnel, in the formal process of constructing federal insurance regulations, or in requests for Medicaid waivers, opponents of health reform were bargaining for a version of the ACA closer to their policy preferences.[4]

How can we account for the variation in how state officials fought back against the reform across the ACA's reform streams?[5] This chapter synthesizes existing literature on the politics of federalism to outline our answer to this question.[6] We argue that although state governments' partisan composition and ideology ultimately shaped their reaction to the ACA overall, how mobilized opponents used US federalism to push back against new reforms depended on three features of the policy context. First, *preexisting policy legacies* (the federal statutes, judicial decisions, and bureaucratic relationships that predate the passage of a law) can alter the incentives opponents have to engage in particular forms of political combat. When new policies build upon strong preexisting legacies of state and federal policy, opponents may find it difficult to use state governments as tools for dissent and may instead look for points of leverage in quiet, intergovernmental bargaining.

Second, opponents may have different opportunities to engage in contestation depending on the extent to which policies *fragment* decision-making authority. When new reforms necessitate action from governors and state legislatures to change the status quo, or when federal officials are given fewer means to coerce or persuade states to comply with policy, opponents may be more likely to engage in outright dissent, refusing to implement federal policy or using state governments' standing in federal court to litigate against the federal government. In contrast, when federal reform can be implemented without legislatures or governors acting to change the status quo, or when the federal government gains the capacity to impose punishments on (or hold back rewards from) uncooperative state governments, opponents may wish to engage in the intergovernmental negotiation of consent.

Finally, we argue that *public sentiments* (public awareness of and support for a reform) can also matter for how postreform politics plays out in the federal system. As a policy's visibility increases and support narrows, its opponents may find it easier to translate the reform into a matter of public debate, whether through state legislative action to contest the reform, litigation against federal agencies, or rhetorical challenges by state officials. As salience declines and public support increases, opponents may be more likely to engage in low-profile intergovernmental bargaining.

The chapter proceeds as follows. We first place the ACA in broader perspective by discussing its similarities to many other public policies in the United States, where authority fragments along the jurisdictional lines of the federal system. Next, we define postreform politics in the context of US federalism by focusing on state governments' consent in policy implementation as well as the construction of political dissent at the state level. We then outline our argument on how institutional fragmentation, public sentiments, and policy legacies shape postreform politics. Finally, we discuss the three policy contexts (health insurance exchanges, Medicaid expansion, and regulatory reform) nested within the ACA, along with the methodological approach we will use to investigate patterns of intergovernmental contestation.

FEDERALISM AS A BATTLEFIELD

Although the ACA, in its attempt to expand access to health insurance is unique in many ways, at least one aspect of its political and institutional context is familiar. The context is US federalism: the constitutional division of sovereignty between the national government and state governments. Federalism, as David Brian Robertson puts it, is an "opportunistic political battlefield with ambiguous boundaries" that make it possible for political battles to take the form of turf wars, with interest groups, political parties, and officials in different jurisdictions (local, state, and federal) fighting over who has the authority to undertake which specific activities.[7]

The politics of turf often displace conflicts over the *substance* of policy; instead of fighting over the federal minimum wage, for example, actors debate whether it is appropriate to set such a wage at the federal level.[8] Even so, political actors rarely fight over turf for its own sake. Winning turf means winning the ability to shape policy to suit your own preferences.[9]

Because the constitutional boundaries for federal and state control are especially ambiguous, federal courts have long been a site of turf wars with high policy stakes. *McCulloch v. Maryland* (1819), for example, established that the federal government had implied powers, not simply powers specified by the Constitution.[10] With the power of the federal government to maintain a national bank hanging in the balance, the stakes in *McCulloch* were high indeed.

Courts are not the only sites for turf wars over federalism. Since the late 1930s, for example, judicial interpretations of the interstate commerce clause of the Constitution have permitted Congress a much broader use of its legislative powers.[11] Yet these decisions did not result in unrestrained centralization of power.[12] Rather, federalism permits political adversaries within Congress to further dispute which level of government should exert influence on its policies. In 1996, opponents of Aid to Families with Dependent Children (AFDC), a social program that supplemented incomes for poor households, successfully turned the program into a block grant to states called Temporary Assistance to Needy Families (TANF). By replacing the AFDC's "entitlement" with TANF's more decentralized block grants and lifetime benefit limits (five years), adversaries were seeking substantive ends. In particular, they hoped more conservative state governments would make social payments conditional on an individual's participation in the labor force.[13]

One reason the division of turf matters so much to litigants, lawmakers, and other political actors is that it provides a staging ground for political conflict after major institutional decisions have been made. When Congress passes a law or the Supreme Court makes a decision, they often reshuffle the "rules of the game" by distributing power to new actors and institutions.[14] Because Congress empowered both state and federal governments to make important decisions related to the ACA's implementation, gaining control of state government meant gaining the ability to shape the outcome of the law. As the next section shows, that division of authority has become crucial to the ACA's *postreform politics*.

WAGING POSTREFORM POLITICS IN THE FEDERAL SYSTEM

In the United States, the passage of a landmark law is a momentous occasion often marked by a sometimes celebratory, sometimes solemn presidential signing ceremony. When the ACA was signed into law in March 2010, photos of the president's signature itself went viral almost immediately, making the legislation itself an icon of his administration's success.[15] If for no other reason, bill signings are historic because passing substantial policy reform is an uphill battle in the United States, beset with challenges from multiple congressional committees and executive agencies, a barrage of interest groups, and members of two legislative chambers.[16]

However worthy of ceremony in its own right, a legislative enactment does not mean the end of political conflict. The implementation of federal reforms on the ground, as Jeffrey Pressman and Aaron Wildavsky's classic 1973 study reminds us, is often a story of how actors with multiple, competing goals can delay, modify, scale down, or otherwise change a law in ways its congressional authors might not have intended.[17] Yet, especially in a climate of intense interest-group opposition and partisan polarization, the politics of implementation involves more than competing visions for an ideal policy. Rather, it often concerns the political legitimacy of the reform itself. As Patashnik puts it, opponents of broad-based reforms, often those who bear their economic costs, "do not disappear after the reforms are passed and may be joined by new clienteles who would also profit from the reforms' unraveling."[18]

Postreform politics owes much to how groups organize after major reforms are passed. If opponents of a reform are well organized, they have a number of options for launching political challenges even after the reform has passed Congress. However, postreform politics also depends on how opponents leverage alternative political *venues*, such as the bureaucracy and the courts, to shape political and policy debates.[19] Federalism thus dramatically expands the menu of options for those waging postreform politics. By dividing authority between levels of government, the US federal system enables actors to engage in political contests over national reforms by taking control of state government. As we will see in Chapter 2, state electoral contests in 2010 became especially competitive and yielded an important "backlash" to the ACA.

Federalism enables opponents of national reforms to engage in two important, but different, forms of political contestation that we will explore in this book.[20] First, federalism creates opportunities for renegotiating—rather than repealing or obstructing—policies after they are made. Because Congress tends to write laws that divide authority between the federal government and the states, those who wish to amend federal laws may lobby state governments for favorable rules.[21] Dividing authority can allow political actors to renegotiate the terms of policy over time, either through intergovernmental bargaining or the application of implementation procedures that differ substantially from state to state.[22] We refer to this process as the *negotiation of consent* between the states and the federal government.

For those interested in a bloodier fight, federalism offers still more opportunities. The division of authority between the federal government and the states gives those who wish to launch political debates about an enacted reform no less than fifty platforms for doing so. In state legislatures and governors' offices around the country, opponents of federal policy can also take action to explicitly dissent from federal laws.[23] This may have immediate implications for policy implementation, but it may also raise public discontent and result in a broader push for repeal. We call this process the *construction of dissent*.

Both consent and dissent emerge out of strong incompatibility between federal and state policy preferences. Sharp disagreements between actors at the federal and state levels can permit political controversy to persist long past the point of enactment. The sources of that conflict are several. First, and perhaps most significantly, conflict can originate from partisan or ideological conflict.[24] Though political fights start in Congress, they do not always end there. Rather, political parties may not want to give up their agendas after losing one legislative battle. Similarly, when parties win, they are conscious that opposition remains, so they refuse to simply "call it a day." Because parties are organized across the levels of the federal system, they are also capable of coordinating bargaining activity beyond Capitol Hill, in federal agencies and in the states.

A second source of conflict in intergovernmental bargaining is organized interest groups.[25] Like parties, groups are highly motivated to pursue their own agendas, even after legislation they oppose is passed. Their resources and attentiveness to politics, as well as their linkage to multiple levels of government, enable them to pursue intergovernmental bargaining.

Finally, conflict can emerge from the differing institutional prerogatives of state and federal officials themselves.[26] Whether federal agencies and state governments are involved in fights over legislation, they are ultimately the actors responsible for implementation and may have specific technical or political concerns that require more flexibility than federal officials may want to grant. Because federal agencies will face criticism on program flaws from congressional committees and the White House, they are motivated to pursue uniform standards across the fifty states.[27]

When deciding how to engage in political conflict, actors do not have to choose between the politics of consent and dissent. As we will show in subsequent chapters, bargaining often occurs in the shadow of dissent, even when dissent does not eventually emerge. However, because we want to explain differing mixtures of strategies across the components of the ACA, we need to treat dissent and consent separately before we can understand how they work together. In the following sections, we describe the characteristics of each of these processes in more detail. We then consider the political and institutional conditions under which political actors should be more likely to undertake either process.

INTERGOVERNMENTAL BARGAINING AND THE
NEGOTIATION OF CONSENT

Adding up to 906 pages, the ACA was not a model of brevity. Yet the legislation left much unsaid. For the first month after its passage, officials at the Department of Health and Human Services (HHS) spent most of their time simply making sense of how the law's ambiguous language might work in practice.[28] When it came to writing rules for health insurance exchanges, for example, there was a great lack of clarity over how much state flexibility should be allowed in rules governing the design of exchanges and the benefits they offered. Because the law only partially preempted state authority, it did not demand the immediate creation of a nationwide health insurance exchange. Federal intervention was instead a last resort; the ACA invited states to establish health insurance exchanges on their own as long as they met minimum federal requirements. The question on federal health officials' minds was how high the bar should be set for states before the federal government intervened.[29]

How did HHS make sense of the intent of Congress? As directed by the ACA itself, HHS worked in cooperation with state insurance commissioners through the National Association of Insurance Commissioners (NAIC), along with nongovernmental stakeholders, to develop standards for regulating insurance plans offered in the new marketplaces. After the ACA's passage, federal regulators negotiated with White House officials, state governments, and the NAIC to produce a Notice of Proposed Rulemaking on exchanges in July 2010.[30] As Table 1.1 shows, the proposed rule prescribed some form of state flexibility on all but four of the topics it covered. HHS also insisted on further consultation with the NAIC on virtually every aspect of exchange plans, including the design of minimum federal standards on which state governments could agree.

By November, the members of the NAIC had voted to adopt model legislation states could pass to meet what they perceived as minimum requirements. Consultation with states continued throughout 2011 in the form of formal meetings in Washington, DC; phone calls; letters; and HHS visits to state capitals.[31] These meetings and consultations were not window dressing on federal fiats; rather, they formed the basic substance of policy. By the time HHS released its final rule on exchanges, it was saturated with the NAIC's decisions on model legislation and evidence of consultation with the states, including direct responses to harsh critiques

Table 1.1 Continuum of State Flexibility by Topic in Proposed Federal Insurance Regulations

Rule	State Flexibility	State Flexibility with a Federal Floor	Nationwide Standard
Qualified health plan selection process	X		
Network adequacy standards	X		
Marketing standards	X		
Agent and broker role in exchange	X		
Streamlined applications for coverage and eligibility		X	
Accountability and governance structure		X	
Subsidiary and regional exchange standards		X	
SHOP employer/employee choice model		X	
Exchange consumer tools: website; call center		X	
Navigator standards		X	
Requirements for qualified health plan offerings		X	
Essential community providers		X	
Qualified health plan accreditation requirements			X
Enrollment periods			X
Approval of state exchanges			X
Transparency reporting requirements			X

Source: Centers for Medicare and Medicaid Services, Presentation on Affordable Insurance Exchanges, State Exchange Grantee Meeting, September 19–20, 2011.

from states that opposed standards they viewed as too exacting.[32] As Chapter 3 will reveal, the negotiation process did not end there.

Why Negotiate Consent?

This brief sketch of the ACA's early weeks and months reveals that when legislative politics end, a new set of conflicts begins. When legislation divides authority between federal and state governments, there is often a struggle between state and federal officials over the terms of public policy itself. Because Congress is often unwilling to give federal agencies the resources necessary to implement policy goals themselves or the authority to direct traffic at the state level, implementation depends on gaining the consent of state and local governments.[33] Thus, those who wish to keep political debate going can, to their great advantage, become involved in the intergovernmental negotiation of consent.[34]

Consent, as opposed to coercion, is a dance for two. In the dance, actors at both levels of government have an incentive to be the leading partner, with more capacity to control policy outcomes—a divergence of preferences that opponents of federal policy can exploit. For both partners, federal and state, the challenge involves finding sources of leverage that allow for their preferences to be met while neither conceding important issues nor risking the erosion of the relationship through refusing to make sacrifices.[35]

Because congressional committees place officials at federal agencies on the hook for failing to implement policy to satisfy their tastes, these officials typically want to ensure that states abide by rules they believe are appropriate to meet policy goals.[36] If the policy goal is improved regulation of workplace safety, federal agencies may want to ensure that all states abide by rules prescribing the regular inspection of factory floors and detailed reviews of employer plans for protecting worker safety, thereby avoiding scrutiny from Congress, whose members control agency budgets.[37] In the case of immigration policy, federal agencies may seek uniform border control by incentivizing particular policing techniques at the local level.[38]

Similarly, state governors, legislatures, and administrative agencies are also motivated to seek control over the terms of public policy. In the case of workplace safety policy, for instance, state governments may want to protect a particularly valuable local industry from costly regulations.[39] With regard to immigration, states with political parties that favor immigrant incorporation may not wish to implement punitive policing techniques for undocumented individuals.[40] Power struggles between federal and state officials may remain dormant or become acrimonious, as we will see in a moment, but the division of authority always creates a possibility for conflict.

To be sure, not all forms of intergovernmental relations involve consent. As Paul Posner shows, Congress also enacts *coercive* regulations, such as direct orders, that place criminal or civil sanctions on state and local governments for not complying with federal regulations on issues such as pollution and fair labor standards, or crossover sanctions used to withdraw federal funding for a federal highway aid program when states fail to abide by regulations on issues such as a minimum drinking age.[41] Although the label "coercive" applies to policies such as these, the extent of coercive intergovernmental relations is often mistakenly used to describe issues over which both federal and state governments have extensive bargaining power. For example, the ACA's insurance exchange provisions are described as coercive because they contain a "partial preemption" rule that allows for the automatic creation of federal insurance exchanges if states do not set up their own. Although these provisions exist, the ACA requires HHS to collaborate with state officials in the design and implementation of standards. Additionally, state governments are not required to spend money on the implementation of exchanges if they do not wish to. So although some elements of the ACA give the federal government added leverage, health reform, like most major reforms passed by Congress, involves a great deal more bargaining than coercion.[42]

The Substance of Intergovernmental Bargaining

To understand intergovernmental bargaining, we first have to consider the items on offer.[43] For any given reform, federal and state governments bargain over a multitude of specifics that, when taken together, dwarf the ACA in terms of length. To make our job easier, we zero in on four major foci of intergovernmental bargaining: *grants, primary authority, waivers,* and *individual regulations.*

Perhaps the most recognizable focus of intergovernmental bargaining is *grants in aid* to states.[44] To encourage states to adopt reforms, Congress often creates voluntary grant programs that provide financial inducements for specific policies. To illustrate just how dominant intergovernmental grants are, a 2010 survey of state finances found that one out of every three dollars of revenue in state budgets came from a federal grant.[45] With this level of federal contribution to state resources, there is much at stake on both sides of the equation. Federal agencies managing policy, as well as Congress and executive organizations such as the Office of Management and Budget (OMB), are understandably concerned about whether states are giving them a satisfactory return on investment.[46] Thus they may desire more stringent requirements on the distribution of funds.

With a large number of federal grant dollars flowing into states, and with the possibility that accepting those dollars involves a sacrifice of control, state governments are also keen on protecting their autonomy to administer grants as they see fit.[47] Especially when the policy goals of state-level political majorities are out of sync with those of federal agencies, states may seek a wide berth and a high level of discretion over grant spending. The central contest in grant bargaining concerns how tightly the federal government can define its policy goals and how far states can push these limits. In the case of the Elementary and Secondary Education Act of 1965 (ESEA), Congress severely curtailed federal government control over the states. Under the law's loose initial arrangement, state and local education agencies had wide latitude and used grant monies to accomplish a variety of goals, many of which were not entirely in keeping with the spirit of the law.[48]

A second focus of intergovernmental bargaining involves which level of government takes *primary authority* in implementing public policy. Primary authority refers to which level of government *directly* implements public programs. When the federal government partially preempts the states' authority, it typically sets conditions under which states can take over the direct administration of programs in lieu of federal control. In partial preemption statutes, Congress or federal administrative agencies permit states to have primary authority for implementing a policy *only* if they can demonstrate that their implementation plans meet minimum federal standards.[49] As we saw earlier, this is precisely the way Congress styled the ACA's provisions for health insurance exchanges.

Though preemption statutes may seem coercive at first, a deeper look at how they work in practice reveals that, as with grants in aid, they involve the politics of bargaining and consent. Because federal officials and the enacting policy coalition may want states to jump through numerous hoops before taking primary authority, states participating in notice-and-comment sessions on federal standards often push for a lower threshold.[50] As with grants, this push often comes not just from opponents within state government but also from interest groups from across the political spectrum that oppose federal policy goals and desire exemptions that apply to the states in which they are highly mobilized.

However coercive partial preemption statutes may appear, they do permit political battles to continue even after policy enactment. In particular, they allow state governments and other interested parties to contest how stringent their implementation plans must be before receiving the federal government's approval. In the 1970s, Congress passed a number of partial preemption statutes to regulate workplace health and safety as well as environmental quality.[51] Statutes such as the Surface Mining Control and Recreation Act and the Occupational Safety and Health Act gave the federal government new powers but also left open the possibility of political bargaining and negotiation between the federal government and the states. This would become crucial to the evolution of policy. A decade after their passage, as a result of protest from the states and from interest groups representing industrial firms, the Reagan administration both decreased federal oversight by shuttering federal field offices and changed the standards for primary authority, granting states more control over these programs.[52]

A third focus of bargaining involves federal *waivers*. In a number of federal laws, Congress allows the states to deviate from federal standards via waivers.[53] When statutes contain waiver provisions (usually for a handful of specific policy goals), federal agencies develop rules and processes whereby states can request the authority to carry out alternative approaches to implementation. After states send in their applications, federal agencies determine whether to grant the waiver. When waivers are rejected, federal agencies typically make a series of recommended revisions, which, if pursued, may lead to approval.[54]

Intergovernmental waiver bargaining is often time-intensive, with many rounds of consultation and negotiation occurring over several years before final approval occurs. Unlike grant bargaining, which involves negotiating how funds will be used, and primary-authority bargaining, which involves the conditions under which states take responsibility for programs, waiver bargaining involves negotiating on more specific details of policy implementation, such as broadening the pool of citizens eligible for a program or using alternative models of financing or administering public policy. In many cases, states may desire waivers for more or less technical reasons in order to experiment with new modes of service provision or to deal with regionally specific policy problems. To the extent that federal officials do not perceive these kinds of waiver requests as conflicting with program goals, they may be more willing to permit them with little fuss.[55] However, as Chapter 4 will show, states do not always seek waivers out of a desire to make incremental adjustments while staying true to a program's goals. Rather, states can seek waivers because of political objections to federal regulations. This raises the stakes of waiver bargaining, because state deviations may ultimately distort how a program functions in ways that challenge what Congress and the bureaucracy hope to achieve. In these cases, bargaining may be more protracted, even to the point of political discord.

A good example of waiver bargaining concerns state experimentation with the Medicaid program under section 1115 of the Social Security Act (SSA).[56] In the early 1990s, many state governments began to focus on improving the health status of low-income residents, many of whom were not covered by Medicaid. To deal with this problem, states requested waivers to redesign their Medicaid programs to include new beneficiaries and shift other beneficiaries from fee-for-service plans toward managed care.[57] Though the George H. W. Bush administration was reluctant to grant these waivers, the Clinton administration was sympathetic to states' policy goals and bargained over state Medicaid adjustments, fifty-six of which were ultimately approved. Without making formal changes to legislation, the political forces for expanding Medicaid then used waivers to permit state experimentation through broadening the program's constituency.[58]

Finally, intergovernmental bargaining can focus on individual program standards established by the federal government. Because the structure of many federal programs depends on states to perform a variety of implementation tasks, states become invested in the details of policy. By implementing policy, states gain technical expertise and tacit knowledge; citizens and interest groups may also begin to perceive states as actors with a legitimate right to make policy decisions.[59] Increased legitimacy and expertise may give states "skin in the game" and thus an incentive to bargain over federal rules outside of grant, authority, and waiver processes.[60] Such negotiations may involve informal dialogues with federal officials, formal participation in notice-and-comment hearings, and congressional hearings on revisions to existing legislation.[61]

This final focus of bargaining is highly heterogeneous, involving negotiations about the mountains of diverse regulations produced by federal agencies. Consider the example of intergovernmental bargaining over federal regulations on

Supplemental Security Income (SSI) after the Social Security Act Amendments of 1972.[62] Though these amendments made the federal government responsible for creating policies that supported the incomes of the aged, blind, and disabled, states successfully contested federal standards for enrollee eligibility and payment procedures. After a long battle, the Social Security Administration eventually approved virtually every variation in standards that states requested, such that the new "centralized" SSI program looked almost identical to the decentralized one that existed prior to 1972. Although Congress did not anticipate this kind of bargaining, it was nevertheless central to postreform politics.[63]

Sources of Leverage

The cases described above reveal several sources of bargaining leverage for opponents of federal reform. First, opponents at the state level gain leverage whenever Congress either writes vague legislation or gives federal agencies poor enforcement and oversight capacities, as we saw in the case of ESEA. Opponents also gain leverage, as we will see in Chapter 3, when federal reforms necessitate action by state legislatures and governors to change the status quo. In so doing, Congress gives states the opportunity to rely on the "will of the people" as a means to challenge decisions of federal agencies. A third source of leverage opponents have is their indispensable capacity to implement programs. As in the case of SSI, states may be able to credibly claim that, without sensible adaptations to their local needs, policy implementation would fail.

STATE GOVERNMENTS AND THE CONSTRUCTION OF DISSENT

For some intense opponents of federal legislation, striking a bargain through intergovernmental negotiation only serves to further entrench an agreement they already find unacceptable. To these actors, bargaining signifies a willingness to cave in. Because these groups and individuals see their ultimate goal as repeal or large-scale retrenchment, they typically engage in a politics of *dissent*.[64]

As with intergovernmental bargaining, dissent often emerges from incompatibilities between partisan, ideological, interest-group, or state-federal preferences. Yet dissent looks much different in practice than negotiated consent. To explore this, let us return for a moment to the case of implementing the ACA's health insurance exchanges. Just as intergovernmental bargaining was heating up in notice-and-comment sessions, another kind of conflict was on the rise that made even the most heated notice-and-comment sessions seem downright collegial. Within a few short months of the law's passage, conservative interest groups and the Virginia attorney general, Ken Cuccinelli, filed lawsuits in federal district court challenging both the law's individual mandate provision as an impermissible use of the commerce power and the expansion of the Medicaid program as an impermissible use of the spending clause.[65] In December, at least one federal judge sided with the law's opponents, and by January 2011, twenty-seven states had signed on to lawsuits challenging HHS over ACA implementation. The case would eventually reach the Supreme Court.[66]

The initial slate of legal challenges proved only partially successful. In June 2012, the Supreme Court upheld the mandate while permitting states to refuse expanding Medicaid.[67] Undeterred, the ACA's opponents continued to push the issue in electoral contests around the country, making it a top domestic issue from the state level to the presidential election.[68] Although Republicans' 2012 presidential hopes—and therefore the promise of a quick repeal of the ACA—were dashed, the contest raged on. The NAIC's model exchange legislation languished and died before reaching the floor in many state legislatures.[69] Republican governors pledged "not to lift a finger" to aid in implementation, leaving federal officials the sizable challenge of designing operable insurance exchanges for a much larger population than they had intended, and on a shoestring budget at that. In short, the ACA's institutional fragmentation and the structure of US federalism itself gave opponents a means of constructing dissent.

Why Construct Dissent?

For those groups or individuals interested in prolonging political debate without sacrificing on core policy concerns, dissent provides an alternative to intergovernmental bargaining. By definition, dissent is not for everyone. Because, as we will see, dissent can be costly and uncertain, actors with moderate or weak policy preferences may be unlikely to engage in it. Although policy opponents engaged in intergovernmental negotiations may wish to simply weaken a law, hopefully to the point of obsolescence, those engaged in dissent may hold stronger preferences and may therefore try to either actively *resist* or *reverse* policy.

What do dissenters hope to achieve? Several major strategies are worth mentioning. First, their actions may be instrumental in eradicating or resisting something obnoxious beyond accommodation. If dissenters truly believe a policy is bad for them, the groups or individuals they represent, or society at large, they may see negotiation or accommodation as unacceptable.[70] Consider the example of a gay-rights group negotiating over the terms of a federal ban on gay marriage. To strong opponents of the ban, pushing for modest accommodations to the Defense of Marriage Act to permit hospital visits for the legally unwedded may look like tacit complicity rather than incremental progress.

Second, individuals with views that fall to the extreme on a given issue may view dissenting activity not as a prelude to outright resistance or repeal but as a source of leverage in intergovernmental bargaining and public persuasion.[71] For extreme opponents of the ACA, bargaining with HHS over minimum federal requirements may shift its outcome decisively in their direction if a prolonged period of dissent and public derision places the federal government in a weakened position in which officials are desperate for states to take on exchange implementation at any cost. Continued dissent may also mean continued public attention to an issue. Even if it does not lead to repeal, continued discussion of the ACA as an illegitimate law only begrudgingly accepted may maintain momentum for scaling it back in the future, or at least for leading policy makers to think twice before adopting similar measures in other policy sectors. So, though the practice of dissent is distinct from negotiating consent, it may ultimately be used as a means to drive harder bargains.

Finally, dissent may serve a purpose that has less to do with dissenters' policy preferences and more to do with their desire for elected office.[72] High levels of partisan conflict can come from sources other than entrenched interest groups. For instance, when competitive elections put parties and political factions such as the Tea Party within reach of controlling Congress, they may have strong incentives to embarrass each other by strategically disagreeing with their policy proposals, thereby ensuring legislative defeat. By refusing to bargain and exercising dissent, opponents of the ACA in Congress or in state governments may hope to edge out electoral competition.

The Substance of Dissent

State dissent from federal reforms is an enduring institutional legacy of US federalism. Since the earliest days of the Republic, long before the emergence of a strong national government, states provided viable venues for national parties to stage political contests over federal policies they opposed.[73] The substance of dissent ranges from litigation and legislation, to quasilegal nullification maneuvers, to political rhetoric and stagecraft. Their differences aside, these techniques share the goal of allowing political battles to continue, even when Washington has taken decisive action. These tools trade off the low cost, collegiality, and relatively certain (if modest) outcomes of intergovernmental bargaining with the possibility of a larger political victory.

First, as we saw above, state-level opponents can engage in litigation on a range of issues. State litigation against the federal government is by no means new. For example, southern states routinely litigated against the federal government on issues related to desegregation.[74] As partisan polarization has increased, however, state attorneys general (AGs) have increasingly coordinated with one another (often along partisan lines) to contest federal legislation and executive actions.[75] Litigation, however, is not limited to Republican AGs or issues of state sovereignty. During the presidency of George W. Bush, Democratic AGs strongly criticized the administration for "regulatory gaps" in drug and financial regulation and sued in federal court to demand stronger enforcement activity.[76] Since 2008, there has been a particularly large spike in multistate AG challenges to federal government activity, a substantial percentage of which feature some form of partisan or ideological coordination.[77]

A second set of tools for constructing dissent includes decisive actions by state legislatures to refuse to cooperate with federal law.[78] Though this practice has taken many forms with varying legal status, it has a long history in the US polity. In 1798, Virginia and Kentucky, hotbeds of opposition to the national government, passed legislative resolutions opposing the Federalist Party's controversial Alien and Sedition Acts. These resolutions claimed that because the Constitution was the result of a "compact" among state governments, the states had the right to interpret the Constitution and declare any laws null and void.

Though the "compact theory" has died innumerable deaths in the courts, its animating idea lives on in state legislation and in amendments that challenge federal law by way of the Constitution.[79] States can pass statutes that affirm a state's nonparticipation in federal programs. Western states with large immigrant populations objected to various federal rules on state drivers' licenses contained in the 2005 REAL ID Act. Doing so was not cheap: states took the risk that their citizens would not be able to use state licenses to board flights.[80] Because of the high costs, nonparticipation is not always pursued for its own sake. Rather, especially when the costs are high, states use nonparticipation to raise the salience of political issues. For instance, state statutes announcing nonparticipation in the REAL ID program explicitly argued that the legislation was designed to "protest the treatment of the states . . . as agents of the federal government" and to lead other state legislatures to do so.[81] A heightened sense of public opposition allowed the states to bargain with the administration over the terms of the act's implementation.

More commonly and consequentially, however, states can engage in dissent by simply failing to cooperate with federal policy. Because the state legislative process is complicated and cumbersome, building a coalition for a dissenting action can be difficult. States opposed to crafting more extensive occupational safety and health laws in the 1970s simply refused to conform themselves to the guidelines of the Occupational Safety and Health Act of 1971. In doing so, they triggered federal preemption of their authority. Yet because the cost of failing to implement new health and safety laws was low, many state governments were willing to engage in "dissent by inaction."[82]

A final way in which states can foment dissent involves deploying the rhetoric of state sovereignty. Whatever the legal status of the "compact theory" may be, the language of nullification still pervades conservative political discourse in the speeches of governors, state legislators, and even US presidents.[83] In 1996, the Republican Party Platform suggested that Democrats had neglected the "solemn compact" of the Tenth Amendment in aggrandizing federal power.[84] These rhetorical moves often have underwritten legislation that takes power away from Washington and moves it to the states, such as the Personal Responsibility and Work Opportunity Reconciliation Act (PRWORA), commonly known as welfare reform.[85] The recent history of state protest over the 2001 No Child Left Behind Act (NCLB) also reveals that there is often no applause line better in state capitals than a critique of tone-deaf Washington bureaucrats insensitive to the needs of teachers, children, and local communities alike.[86] Though such appeals are unlikely to result in the repeal of federal laws, they do place issues on the agenda that would not be there otherwise, often with the hope of scoring political points for negotiating with the federal government.

Sources of Leverage

As the discussion above suggests, political actors who wish to use state-level institutions to pursue a strategy of dissent depend on several sources of leverage. First, strategies of dissent rely on legal uncertainty.[87] Because dissenters may not want to pay the costs of noncompliance, they need legal and political justification for dissent that allows them to escape without punishment. Such defenses are built on the premise that law is "not yet settled," either because courts have not issued rulings on issues such as constitutionality or because political actors have failed to reach consensus. When the status of a federal law has been formally contested in the courts or is likely to invite legal challenges given the present state of the legal doctrine, states may find it easier to openly contest federal statutes. States may also be more willing to experiment with dissent when federal intervention in a particular field has fewer historical antecedents, which may also raise the specter of illegitimacy. By contrast, as policies receive judicial rulings, additional administrative decisions, and further legislative adjustments, dissenters can no longer claim major issues are "not yet settled," weakening legal justification for dissent as well as its rhetorical appeal.

The political leverage of opponents is also improved when federal policies lower the "costs" of dissent. In particular, federal policies that fragment authority by necessitating new action by state legislatures and governors can make dissent a routine matter. First, dissenters may gain leverage when laws necessitate highly salient decisions to be taken by governors or in political venues such as state legislatures. The ACA invited dissent by creating health insurance exchanges, institutions virtually no states already possessed. This took decisions about the ACA out of an administrative realm and placed them in a potent political arena in which vitriol for "Obamacare" had not yet died down. Second, dissenters benefit from laws that divide administrative authority. As we have seen, the federal-state division of drug enforcement authority allows proponents of state marijuana legalization to dissent from enforcement without fearing a large federal crackdown. Finally, dissenters benefit from federal laws that lower the cost of dissenting activity. When there are no federal prohibitions on dissent, or when dissent does not invite an especially costly fiscal or legal penalty such as the REAL ID flight ban, states may find it easier to dissent or, if the goal is bargaining, threaten to do so. Similarly, when states judge "rewards" of participation, including the size of federal grants, to be minimal, dissent may become a more attractive option.

A third source of leverage is public opinion skeptical toward federal reform. When public sentiments on an issue are not in favor of a federal policy, as in the case of NCLB, state governments may enjoy deference from the federal government, even if their actions are legally suspect. Though federal officials at the Bureau of Alcohol, Tobacco, and Firearms (ATF) may be suspicious of state "firearm freedom" legislation that opposes federal weapon regulations, they may not want to invite a swirl of public hostility for stepping in to invalidate intrastate firearms sales in Montana. The ideal situation for political opponents is *mass opposition* to a federal reform, but this is not strictly necessary. Dissenting states may benefit greatly when they can show that an issue, the legalization of marijuana for instance, is "gaining ground" in public opinion. In this case, they suffer little risk of punishment—either in the form of federal sanctions or electoral blame—for refusing to cooperate with federal reforms. By contrast, when public sentiments are firmly in favor of a federal policy goal—consider the prevention of a terrorist attack in the wake of the September 11, 2001, attacks—states may be less able to provide a reasonable public justification for actively opposing US Department of Homeland Security policies. Not only might governors or state legislators face electoral punishments for raising objections but also public opinion gives federal agencies greater leverage to impose sanctions.

OUR ARGUMENT: HOW POLICY LEGACIES, INSTITUTIONAL FRAGMENTATION, AND PUBLIC SENTIMENTS SHAPE POSTREFORM POLITICS

The discussion thus far reveals that each form of postreform politics in the federal system, consent and dissent, may be more likely to emerge in some circumstances than others. One rather obvious set of factors is opponents' specific goals and the intensity of their preferences.[88] State administrators who oppose federal reform but are engaged in long-standing patterns of intergovernmental negotiation may wish to continue this pattern, either because they have political beliefs that align with those of federal administrators that make intergovernmental bargaining a natural choice or because of social or professional interests in keeping up cordial ties with federal agencies.[89] In contrast, for reasons reflecting policy preferences, partisanship, ideology, interest-group ties, or an effort to build a reputation with the electorate, state legislators and governors may find dissent a more natural strategy.

Though political actors' ideas, goals, and preferences help us situate their willingness to use particular strategies, they alone are not sufficient for understanding how actors decide on strategy. Even actors with extreme political preferences, for instance, may not be able to exercise dissent when they do not have access to the decision-making process or when the costs of resistance are too high. We argue instead that political and institutional contexts dramatically affect the incentives actors have to engage in each type of strategy. As we will show in subsequent chapters, there are three contextual factors that matter most for shaping the politics of federalism: *policy legacies, institutional fragmentation,* and *public sentiments.*

Policy Legacies

A first factor that can influence postreform politics is the *policy legacy* that exists prior to the adoption of a new reform.[90] The term refers to the preexisting pattern of federal legislation, judicial rulings, and intergovernmental relationships in a particular area of governance, such as the establishment of health insurance markets, health insurance for the poor, or market regulation. As the complexity of this definition reveals, legacies are made up of many working parts, but their differences can be more easily summarized along a continuum in terms of their "thickness."

Thick policy legacies contain extensive prior federal and state action on an issue, with large budgetary commitments; rulings from higher federal courts, including the Supreme Court, that uphold the legality of these actions; and deep working relationships between federal and state governments, with routine interaction and negotiation. A good example of a thick policy legacy is that of contemporary legislation governing air pollution. Since the 1960s, Congress has passed numerous federal and state statutes concerning air pollution; these statutes have been roundly upheld in federal courts and are administered by intergovernmental networks of policy professionals.[91]

Thin policy legacies, in contrast, feature minimal legislation, few judicial rulings, and little intergovernmental interaction. A good example of a thin policy legacy is that of law governing hydraulic fracturing (fracking).[92] Fracking has as yet failed to generate strong regulatory frameworks in the states. Federal legislation does not exist, nor do many federal court decisions on the legality of such policy. Federal-state collaboration on fracking governance is minimal and lacks efficacy. As states and federal agencies begin to consider fracking more seriously, the fracking policy legacy could thicken, with more comprehensive legislation, judicial tests, and networks of policy professionals emerging slowly over time.

Depending on how thick a policy legacy is, postreform politics may bend toward the construction of dissent or the negotiation of consent. First, policy legacies may encourage political opponents to mobilize their resources toward different ends. When policy legacies are particularly thick, with recognizable legislation at the state and federal level upheld by courts and supported by preexisting intergovernmental networks, even mobilized opponents may find it to their advantage to engage in the negotiation of consent. For example, if the federal government is more than willing to use standards for air quality developed in collaboration with state governments as federal minimums, opponents may have strong incentives to be "at the table" rather than "on the menu" when those standards are set or to push for waivers from those standards after they are on the books.[93] In contrast, when policy legacies are especially thin, with few antecedent laws, questionable constitutional status, and little history of intergovernmental collaboration on the policy, dissent, whether in the form of a refusal to take part in a reform, litigation, or lobbying, may make more strategic sense for opponents.[94]

Policy legacies may also shape the success of political strategies after opponents begin to pursue them. Opponents pursuing dissent in the form of litigation when there is an especially clear history of judicial affirmation of the policy in question may be assuming more risk and may therefore choose to mix their strategy with intergovernmental bargaining.[95] Similarly, opponents may find it difficult to effectively pursue state legislative action challenging a federal reform when state administrative agencies have implemented similar reforms in the past. When policy legacies are contested, such as when there are some similar federal policies and conflicting judicial rulings, opponents of federal policy may be more likely to mix strategies of consent and dissent.

Institutional Fragmentation

The second factor that matters in explaining postreform politics in the federal system is institutional fragmentation, or the extent to which decision-making authority is divided between governmental institutions. On the *highly fragmented* end of the continuum, Congress designs public policies that necessitate *state legislative approval* (usually from state legislatures and governors).[96] Though federal legislation rarely refers to state legislatures specifically, state legislative approval is necessary most often when federal programs give states the opportunity to establish *new* policies.[97] With high fragmentation, the federal government also possesses fewer tools of coercion, such as fines or penalties, and may lack the capacity to step in if states refuse to cooperate. The ACA's provisions on insurance exchanges are highly fragmented because they both necessitate action by state legislatures and governors to create exchanges and impose few punishments on states for not doing so.

On the *unfragmented* end of the continuum, Congress can make state involvement more inconsequential. It can do so by allowing state agencies to implement federal reforms under the authority they already have, requiring no additional action by state legislatures. Some partial preemption statutes, for example, give the federal government a great deal of capacity to step in if states fail to establish programs that meet minimum standards and do not necessitate extensive approval by state legislatures.[98] In the middle of the continuum are policies that contain punishments for states that do not cooperate but still necessitate action by state legislatures and governors to implement reform. The Occupational Safety and Health Act, for instance, imposed penalties on states for noncooperation but necessitated more extensive action by state legislatures and governors by setting out specific new regulations with which states had to comply in order to implement reforms.[99]

Increased institutional fragmentation incentivizes the construction of dissent, whereas a lower level of fragmentation promotes the negotiation of consent.[100] There are two reasons why. First, when states must take more extensive action to implement federal reforms, opponents gain leverage because of the low cost of dissent. If state legislatures must act to change the status quo, opponents can more easily stall cooperative activity through restricting the passage of new legislation. Conversely, less fragmented policies may create fewer opportunities for influence. When state agencies can implement federal policies under their existing authority, this requires opponents to build a legislative coalition to restrict that authority. The veto points of the state legislative process can work *against* dissent in these cases. Even if interest groups have access to state administrative agencies, it may be difficult for them to preclude negotiation between federal and state governments in favor of dissent.

Second, institutional fragmentation may also affect opponents' *incentives* to engage in dissent. Especially high levels of fragmentation may induce actors to engage in dissent for two reasons. When federal officials have fewer coercive tools, this may lower the costs of dissent.[101] For example, if the federal government does not have the institutional capacity to impose sanctions or take retaliatory measures for dissenting actions, it may signal that resistance or noncooperation for its own sake will go unchallenged. When federal agencies have greater coercive capacity, dissent for its own sake may be less attractive to opponents than inter-governmental negotiation, assuming they can gain access to administrative venues in which negotiation occurs. In these circumstances, even extreme political opponents may find that intergovernmental bargaining can result in some concrete gains at a much lower "price."

Fragmentation may also allow states to credibly *threaten* dissent as a means to harder bargaining.[102] This is especially true when states must take action to implement new policies and when federal officials have little capacity to step in if states do not act. By contrast, when federal officials *can* impose sanctions for non-compliance or have sufficient resources for policy implementation in the absence of state actions, states' threats of noncooperation become less meaningful and may be highly ineffective. As a result, political conflict may take the form of negotiated consent.

Public Sentiments

A final crucial factor is the character of *public sentiments* on federal policy. Public sentiments refer to the normative assumptions that constrain political elites by limiting the range of decisions they are likely to see as appropriate.[103] We can characterize public sentiments according to two dimensions: *issue salience* and *public support* for a federal policy. Issue salience is the extent to which broad public and interest group audiences recognize an issue of federal policy as important.[104] High salience issues of federal policy tend to either directly affect broad swaths of citizens (e.g., taxes) or evoke meaningful political or cultural symbols, even if their effects on most individuals are minimal (e.g., legislation prohibiting flag burning).

Public *support* for federal policy refers to the popularity of a policy with mass audiences.[105] When public support for an issue is high, we should see solid majorities or supermajorities of public approval in a broad cross section of polling data. Low public support is indicated by widespread public disapproval. Finally, mixed public support is indicated by roughly comparable levels of public approval and disapproval.

Both issue salience and public support matter as opponents try to exercise leverage in the federal system. First, issue salience can shape how actors opposed to federal policy decide how to invest their time and effort. Because dissent-oriented strategies often require a baseline level of public concern, opponents may not wish to use these strategies when issue salience is low. Though dissent-oriented political strategies often require *making* issues salient when they are not already so, some issues have more potential than others.[106] Try as they might, even wizards of political messaging may find it difficult to squeeze salience out of technically complex regulatory policies with little direct effect on the public. Instead, opponents of these policies may have better luck with a strategy that relies on intergovernmental negotiation.

When issue salience is higher, public *support* for federal policy begins to matter. High levels of public support create incentives for intergovernmental bargaining. In the case of homeland-security policy in the immediate aftermath of the September 11 attacks, high public support for antiterrorism policy may have made it difficult for states to thwart the implementation of PATRIOT Act provisions, whereas intergovernmental bargaining may have been more viable.[107] Within a decade, however, as public support dwindled, it became possible for states to engage in dissent on federal border-control activities.[108]

When public support is mixed or low and issue salience is high, however, opponents may find that intergovernmental bargaining alone insufficient. Low support for federal policy is ideal for dissenters because it may mean that political support exists for any number of assertive actions. Because they benefit from widespread in-state opposition to federal drug policy, proponents of issues such as marijuana legalization have found dissent-oriented strategies successful, with legislative victories in states such as California, Colorado, and Washington. Mixed public support also provides a window of opportunity to challenge federal policy. Opponents of federal education policy in Utah relied on the mixed public feelings over NCLB to generate the passage of legislation that declared the state's intention to prioritize state, rather than federal, education policy directives when the two were in conflict.[109]

Overview of the Argument

We argue that the negotiation of consent in postreform politics in the federal system, especially in the contemporary period of intense partisanship, is more likely to emerge when institutional fragmentation is low, when public sentiments are characterized by low issue salience or high support for federal policy, and when policy legacies are thick. In contrast, postreform politics should tend toward the construction of dissent when institutional fragmentation is high, public sentiments are characterized by high issue salience and low or mixed support for federal policy, and policy legacies are thin. Obviously, variations in policy legacies, institutional fragmentation, and public sentiments may not always track each other, yet our predictions, summarized in Table 1.2, should be especially easy to test when they do.

There is one final point we wish to emphasize. Our argument does not suggest that the politics of consent and dissent are mutually exclusive. Rather, especially when the political and institutional environments give political actors contradic-

Table 1.2 Predicted Effects of Policy Legacy, Institutional Fragmentation, and Public Sentiments

Factor	Definition	Predicted Effect on Negotiation of Consent	Predicted Effect on Construction of Dissent
Policy legacy	The degree to which a policy has historical predecessors at the federal and state level, judicial rulings affirming its legality, and intergovernmental networks of professionals supporting it	+	−
Institutional fragmentation	The degree to which a policy necessitates state decision making and administration and gives the federal government weak coercive capacity	−	+
Public sentiments	The degree of a policy's salience and support	Salience: − Support: +	Salience: + Support: −

tory signals, we expect to find a combination of strategies at work, especially the use of dissent as a threat in intergovernmental bargaining. When the signals are clearer, however, we should expect to find one type of politics or the other.

STUDYING POSTREFORM POLITICS IN THE ACA

Though our analysis is limited to the ACA, the law's complexity and the striking differences in intergovernmental politics demand that we use an explicitly *comparative* approach to study it.[110] Both conventional media and academic studies of the ACA treat it as a single reform, but even a casual glance at the ACA's statutory text reveals that health reform cannot be boiled down to any one element of the law. Rather, the ACA is one large umbrella reform built from many smaller, sometimes unrelated reforms that cover topics as diverse as expanding the health care workforce to improving the quality of coverage for mental health to incentivizing individuals to adopt healthy eating habits. These smaller reforms may affect one another in the long run, but they operate autonomously; each relies on its own institutional setup, political opponents and supporters, and policy legacies. Whether political actors think about these reforms in the aggregate, decisions about them are made separately, with different sets of meetings, stakeholders, regulation, legislation, and judicial decisions. Here, we outline those differences and briefly describe our approach to studying them.

Variation across Major Reforms within the ACA

Although we had our pick of reforms to study, we chose the three most widely seen as substantively significant for health care delivery: *health insurance exchanges*, *Medicaid expansion*, and *regulatory reform*. As the following chapters will show, each of these reforms varies from the others in terms of institutional fragmentation, public sentiments, and policy legacies. Table 1.3 briefly previews the differences between these individual reforms. Each reform, as the following chapters will show, has a unique blend of institutional and political contexts.

The policy differences between exchanges, Medicaid, and regulatory reforms are particularly striking and suggest that although state governments' partisanship and policy preferences help to explain their responses to the ACA, the incentives for consent and dissent varied across the three reforms. First, policy legacies vary widely between the reforms. Prior to the ACA's passage, no federal agency had created health insurance marketplaces, and only Massachusetts had an operable example of what such an exchange would look like. Prior to 2010, there were few judicial tests of the legality of federal health insurance policy—leaving the area wide open to challenge in the courts. For opponents of the ACA in state governments, the potential that the law would be overturned greatly lowered the costs of dissent and made investments increasing state exchanges a riskier proposition. By contrast, the Medicaid program has had a long history of federal-state collaboration and extensive previous action by the federal and state governments on expanding eligibility but still faces some state-federal conflicts and judicial challenges with respect to the legality of federal action. Dissent was thus costlier, and consent more attractive, in states that had legacies of federal-state collaboration, even if opposition to the ACA ran high. Finally, though the legacy of federal-state collaboration on insurance collaboration is not as long as that of Medicaid, virtually all states gave their insurance commissioners some authority to regulate the insurance market (as opposed to the individual mandate to purchase insurance). This allowed federal agencies to work within existing state frameworks for consumer protection to promote new policy goals, lowering the costs of bargaining and consent even in states with strong opposition to the ACA.

Second, institutional fragmentation varied across the cases. Legislative provisions on health insurance exchanges were highly fragmented. Because few states operated exchanges when the ACA passed, state legislatures and governors had to make political decisions to create institutions that imposed new costs on state

Table 1.3 Patterns and Predictions for the Postreform Politics of the ACA

	Health Insurance Exchanges	Medicaid Expansion	Regulatory Reform
Policy Context			
Policy legacy	thin	mixed	mixed
Institutional fragmentation	high	medium	low
Public sentiments	high salience, mixed support	high salience, mixed support	low salience, support unclear
Predictions for Postreform Politics			
Negotiation of consent	minimal	mixed	extensive
Construction of dissent	extensive	mixed	minimal

government with no clear guarantee of benefits. State governors and legislators opposed to the ACA also faced little punishment for failing to create exchanges because they believed the federal government would set up substitute exchanges and the Internal Revenue Service (IRS) would distribute premium tax credits to individuals on those exchanges. The design of Medicaid expansion is slightly less fragmented. Though the Supreme Court in *National Federation of Independent Business (NFIB) v. Sebelius* has invalidated what it deemed the expansion's coercive provisions, the federal government still retains its ability to provide strong fiscal inducements to the states as well as to hospitals and providers within states to make the expansion. Unlike exchanges, the benefits of consent (and the costs of dissent) on Medicaid are also higher given that governors can set the agenda through the section 1115 waiver process and have historically dominated the Medicaid policy arena. Finally, the design of regulatory reforms for the insurance industry is much less fragmented. Because many states already had regulatory frameworks in place when the ACA passed, and given that federal regulators respected and worked within these frameworks, they could implement federal policy without extensive interference from state legislatures and governors. Thus the costs of dissent were much higher because would-be dissenters would have had to undo existing state consumer-protection rules. Further, the ACA explicitly permits federal officials to preempt the authority of states that do not adhere to new federal rules.

Finally, public sentiments on each of the reforms varied substantially. Whereas Medicaid expansion and insurance exchanges were highly salient to consumers of health insurance (not to mention popular media), regulatory reforms were hardly discussed in press coverage of the ACA. The salience of the first two reforms was also accompanied by sharply divided public support, providing opponents of the ACA leverage for the construction of dissent. By contrast, when public audiences were surveyed about their opinions on regulatory reforms, they tended to respond favorably. Thus turning regulatory reforms into a subject of symbolic politics of dissent would have been difficult for opponents of the ACA to do.

Methodology and Sources of Evidence

Our methodological approach involved a close comparison of institutional fragmentation, public sentiments, and policy legacies across these major components of the ACA.[111] To assess policy legacies, we consulted legislative histories and analyses done by government agencies, prior judicial rulings, and histories of administrative relationships between federal and state agencies. To unpack the institutional design of each reform and more importantly the extent of institutional fragmentation, we examined all relevant provisions of the ACA, all relevant sections of the Supreme Court's ruling in *NFIB v. Sebelius*, and all regulations issued by federal agencies related to exchanges, Medicaid expansion, and regulatory reform. Finally, to analyze public sentiments, we systematically collected pertinent secondary literature, including academic studies and news reports, in an attempt to gather evidence of salience and public support for the federal policy.

In exploring postreform politics, we used two general checklists to guide our collection of data. For evidence of the negotiation of consent, we relied on notice-and-comment proceedings, minutes of intergovernmental meetings, correspondence between officials, and when possible, interviews with officials. We scoured these materials for evidence of negotiation on intergovernmental grants in aid, standards for primary authority, intergovernmental waivers, and specific adjustments to the federal regulations. For evidence of dissent, we conducted broad searches of state legislation and litigation databases as well as news reports containing dissenting rhetoric of state officials. Here, we were looking for evidence of state-driven litigation over the ACA as it traveled through federal courts, state legislation or inaction indicating opposition to various reforms within the ACA, and rhetorical statements indicating states' intention to carry out legislation and litigation that obstructed the ACA's implementation.

Because the ACA is still a law in motion, we limited our analysis of postreform politics to events that occurred between the passage of the reform in March 2010 and the close of open enrollment in April 2014. Beyond the practical reason for this limit (our desire to carry out a study of the ACA), there is a good intellectual justification for examining the early stages of the law's life. However in flux, legislation is typically *path dependent*, meaning early decisions affect the outcome of decisions taken later.[112] For instance, if Republican states refuse to create health insurance exchanges and engage in other acts of dissent, this has downstream consequences for their reputation as "hard bargainers" and could elicit distinctive actions from federal officials in the future. So although we may be limited in postulating long-term political trends in the ACA, the following chapters offer a thorough look at a defining period in the life of this landmark reform. We begin by examining the broader political context in which the implementation of health reform has taken place.

2. Uncertain Victory: The Political Context of Health Care Reform Implementation

For supporters of health care reform, the signing ceremony for the Patient Protection and Affordable Care Act (ACA) in late March 2010 was a moment of jubilation. Having navigated a political minefield that had dogged previous attempts at expanding health insurance in the United States, supporters had cause for excitement. Memorably, Vice President Joe Biden, in what was supposed to be a private remark, was overheard saying, "Mr. President, this is a big fucking deal." President Barack Obama declared that the bill enshrined the "core principle that everybody should have some basic security when it comes to their health care." He further commented that the ACA would "set in motion reforms that generations of Americans have fought for and marched for and hungered to see." Senator Max Baucus (D-MT), another central figure in the legislative process, who served as chair of the Senate Finance Committee, urged Republican opponents to accept the reality of comprehensive health care reform. He said, "Now it is a fact. Now it is law. Now it is history."[1]

Yet Republicans in Congress remained bitterly opposed to the reform, and ideological groups on the right mobilized almost immediately in favor of repeal and constitutional challenges. Furthermore, insurance industry representatives and employers, dissatisfied with many core concepts in the law, prepared to fight over a number of specific provisions Congress had left for federal agencies to decide during the regulatory process. As the 2010 midterm elections came into full swing, opponents of health care reform mobilized to win power not only in Congress but also at the state level, where much of the ACA's implementation would take place. In the states partisan, ideological, and business opponents of the ACA redoubled their efforts to win control of government institutions and contest the reform. Such opposition was well organized and sustained. Six months after President Obama's reelection, which affirmed the expansion of Medicaid and opening the insurance exchanges, Senate Minority Leader Mitch McConnell (R-KY) explained that he and his colleagues would continue to oppose the law. On an episode of NBC's *Meet the Press* in May 2013, McConnell described the ACA as the "single worst piece of legislation that's been passed in modern times in this country" and predicted that the reform would remain a key electoral issue.[2] At that point, conservative opponents of the ACA were happy to quote Senator Baucus, who a month earlier had said, "I just see a huge train wreck coming down."[3]

Nearly a year later, and for the fiftieth time, the Republican-controlled House voted to repeal or alter the ACA.[4] However, the end of March 2014 marked a significant moment in the implementation of the ACA. The rollout of the ACA was hardly complete, but the first period of open enrollment in the newly created health insurance exchanges had drawn to a close, and Medicaid expansion and regulatory regimes in the states were beginning to take shape. The following chapters examine how key opponents of the ACA acted to further their policy preferences, partisan ambitions, and perceived interests in the four years following the signing ceremony. Understanding those developments requires looking back at how the ACA was designed and enacted from 2009 to 2010, which will allow us to identify how the law itself provided incentives for compliance or provided opportunities for opponents to resist its strictures. We focus in particular on the strategies used by the law's opponents to undermine both the institutional foundations of the law and popular support for it.

The overall legislative process culminating in the passage of the ACA has been well documented,[5] but it is important to recognize how the specific details of the law's design encompassed or eliminated potential points of institutional leverage over policy implementation. The more the points of leverage in a law, the more uncertain it is that the law will roll out in practice as intended by its designers. As Eric Patashnik and Julian Zelizer explain, "In American democracy policy entrenchment has limits. . . . Whether a new policy establishes facts on the ground and creates pressure for its own maintenance is an empirical question."[6] As Elizabeth Rigby and her colleagues articulate, it is important to pay proper "attention to fundamental questions of policy design" and understand "politics . . . as a contest over policy—and therefore a contest with durable, substantive, and high stakes for political actors and institutions alike."[7]

The high-voltage politics of passing the ACA, as we illustrate in this chapter, motivated its fiercest opponents to challenge the law's implementation. In particular, we show that the ACA's fragmented structure propelled opponents to mobilize at the state level to slow implementation and to subvert key policy priorities, making state officials—on which we focus in the chapters to come—potential veto points for the reform.[8]

DESIGNING REFORM

With deep-seated problems afflicting the US health care system, the task of devising comprehensive change was highly problematic. Reformers had to expand access to health insurance for millions of Americans at a cost that these mostly low-income households could afford while simultaneously bending the so-called cost curve in order to restrain aggregate spending on health care. For the liberal wing of the Democratic Party, the solution to this dilemma lay to the north in the Canadian single-payer model, which guarantees universal coverage and grants the government a greater capacity to regulate providers and control costs. Although a single-payer system has the beauty of relative simplicity, it was not seen as a politically viable option, in part because of the powerful interests created by the existing public-private health care system, which crystalized during the post–World War II era. In 2003, when first contemplating a run for the US Senate, Obama had claimed to be a "proponent of a single-payer universal health care plan," but as president he and his congressional allies focused on ways of building on the existing health care infrastructure rather than replacing it.[9] It was assumed that most Americans would continue to get their health insurance through employers. That way, the government would focus on increasing levels of assistance to people excluded from the employer-based market as well as tightening regulation of the private insurance market to contain costs. Yet how these objectives would be accomplished was not so obvious. Previous efforts at "stretching and reworking the existing health care system" had "not been a recipe for pain-free consensus."[10] In particular, the Clinton administration's experience in 1993 and 1994 had cast a long shadow, discouraging efforts at comprehensive reform. The events of the early 1990s illustrated how quickly a consensus that a major overhaul of the country's health care arrangements was needed and had public support changed into a consensus that comprehensive reform was impractical and unpopular.

The events of 1993 and 1994 were not encouraging for President Obama and his congressional allies in January 2009. Nevertheless, the new president pressed ahead, even though his chief of staff, Rahm Emmanuel, and Vice President Biden had reservations about simultaneously pursuing economic and health policy reform.[11] However, the new president did in fact have some significant institutional advantages over his Democratic predecessor that boosted the opportunity for passing reform in Congress.[12] Critically, Obama was dealing with bigger and more coherent Democratic majorities in Congress than Clinton had worked with sixteen years earlier.[13] Moreover the "compelling evidence of systemwide problems in health care across the domains of costs, coverage, and consequences" evident in the 1990s had become "even more pronounced" by the late 2000s, adding momentum to the reform train.[14] President Obama also consciously chose to adopt a different legislative strategy than Clinton. While Clinton presented Congress with a "take it or leave it" detailed reform plan, the Obama White House gave general instructions about the final goals but left congressional leaders to devise the details of reform.[15]

Importantly this strategy not only reflected a conscious effort to adopt a different approach than Clinton used but it also indicated an emerging consensus, at least among Democrats, about what reform would look like. In 2009, unlike in 1993, there was now an apparently viable model of how to significantly reduce the number of uninsured and increase a regulatory presence in the insurance market. That model was the Massachusetts law passed in April 2006 by the state's Democratic legislature and signed by its Republican governor, Mitt Romney. Among its provisions, the law expanded the state's Medicaid program to cover more children, created an exchange where adults with incomes up to 300 percent of the poverty level could buy subsidized insurance, introduced an individual mandate, and aimed to make insurance affordable through insurance market reforms.[16] At the signing ceremony, Governor Romney said, "This isn't 100 percent of what anyone in this room wanted. . . . But the differences between us are small."[17] One of the state's Democratic US senators, Edward Kennedy, a long-standing champion of comprehensive reform, added, "You may well have fired the shot heard round the world on health care in America. I hope so."[18]

This success of the Massachusetts bipartisan reform suggested that it might provide a model for national policy. In fact, the state's reform created a prototype that eased access to coverage for low-income households through the creation of a health insurance exchange, which appealed to advocates across the ideological spectrum. Two scholars from the conservative Heritage Foundation noted, with approval, how such a reform had brought about the "reorganization of a large part of the state's private insurance system into a 'single market' structure with uniform rules and a central 'clearinghouse' for administering coverage."[19] From 2006 onward, the Massachusetts principle of the exchange became embedded in ideas about how to expand coverage. Conservatives liked that the state's exchange did not directly involve the government as a provider or purchaser of insurance, which meant that the exchange could be seen as part of an "evolution of a consumer-focused approach to health system change."[20] For liberals, by subsidizing low-income households to purchase insurance, the exchange provided a means of expanding access to insurance for people who might otherwise have gone uninsured. However, not everyone was in agreement that this unique statewide system would map neatly onto the national landscape. Considerable media coverage during the ACA's legislative process focused on a separate idea of a public option whereby the government would offer an insurance package that would compete with private insurers in the exchange. The attention on the public option, however, distracted from another important issue of policy design. The question was: Should there be a national exchange, or should the states create their own institutions? Furthermore, the Massachusetts example also offered only partial answers to national concerns in other policy areas discussed in this book. The state expanded its Medicaid program, but this did not explain how an expansion would be funded across the country, especially in states that had much higher preexisting rates of uninsured than Massachusetts. In addition, increasing regulation of the insurance market was a significant part of the 2006 reform efforts to keep the cost of insurance down in order to maintain affordability. Because Massachusetts already had a relatively tightly regulated insurance market, particularly with regard to the small-group and individual insurance market, the changes made in the state to control premium rate increases did not provide a template that could be easily applied to all states.[21]

Overall, the climate for designing policy was more promising than in 1993, but it was far from settled. The emerging consensus on the principles of how to move forward meant that the new president "didn't need to jump-start or guide the legislative process by drawing up his own bill" because "congressional Democrats already agreed on the direction they were going to take, and it was the same direction that Obama favored."[22] Still, the favorable institutional environment and the agreement on the broad contours of what reform should look like did not guarantee success because the legislative process remained laden with potential veto points.[23] Furthermore, "broad" agreement was just that, with many devilish details to be worked out.

ENACTING REFORM

It became evident to observers that any reform would hinge heavily, if not exclusively, on Democratic electoral support. The new president liked to talk about working in a bipartisan fashion, and in March 2009 more than 150 participants, including some Republican legislators as well as representatives from interest groups who had traditionally aligned against reform, attended a high-profile White House conference to discuss reform.[24] At this stage there was even optimistic talk of a bill to be signed by Thanksgiving of 2009. In May 2009, at another White House event, President Obama declared that the "stars are aligned" for the passage of major reform.[25] Yet all the political figures who gathered with the president on the White House lawn that day were fellow Democrats, though there were efforts at bringing some Republicans on board the reform train. In fact, in the early stages of deliberating how to reach the broad goals the White House outlined, there was some Republican input into the bill. According to political scientists Lawrence Jacobs and Theda Skocpol, "Hundreds of amendments proposed by House or Senate Republicans received enough support to make it into the advancing legislation" with "significant elements of the final legislation . . . shaped by these negotiations."[26] For instance, the Senate Health, Education, Labor, and Pensions Committee bill included more than 160 Republican amendments accepted during the monthlong markup.[27] In the end, however, the final vote in that committee was strictly along party lines.[28] Initial signs of bipartisanship in the Senate Finance Committee (SFC) also failed to endure. The so-called Gang of Six negotiations consisted of three Democrats: SFC chair Max Baucus, who led the negotiations, Jeff Bingaman (New Mexico), and Kent Conrad (North Dakota) as well as three Republicans: Michael Enzi (Wyoming), Olympia Snowe (Maine), and Charles Grassley (Iowa). They met regularly through early summer 2009, with a *New York Times* report predicting, "The fate of the health care overhaul largely rests on the shoulders of six senators."[29] Later in the summer, however, hopes for a compromise were disappearing. In mid-August, Baucus persisted in public displays of optimism, declaring that the SFC was "on track to reach a bipartisan agreement on comprehensive health care reform," but few onlookers shared that perspective.[30] In the end, Senator Snowe did vote for the SFC's version of health care reform, but that was the only vote cast by a Republican senator in favor of reform at any point in the process.

Robust Republican opposition meant that differences within Democratic ranks would need to be reconciled, especially in the Senate, to ward off a filibuster. The most high profile of the Democrats' internal disputes was over the so-called public option. This plan would have put the federal government in competition with private insurers by allowing it to sell health insurance directly to individuals through the insurance exchanges, offering subsidized insurance packages to lower-income households.[31] The final House version did in fact contain a public option provision. In the Senate, where independent Senator Joe Lieberman of Connecticut made it plain he would not vote for any bill with the public option, this stance was effectively killed. President Obama did make public statements supporting the principle of the public option but did not prioritize the idea over securing the passage of a reform bill in the Senate.[32]

The debate over the public option, along with other high-profile disputes over Medicare "death panels" (end-of-life counseling) and possible public funding for access to abortion, took attention away from decision making in other areas of policy design ultimately critical to the ACA's implementation. Although there was general consensus among reformers on the need to expand Medicaid, establish insurance exchanges, and tighten regulation of insurers, there was no automatic agreement on how to accomplish those goals. In deciding how best to structure the Medicaid program, the key questions circled around how generous that expansion should be and, more problematically, how it would be funded. The bill developed in the House settled on coverage for people who earned up to 150 percent of the federal poverty level (FPL) with two years of full federal funding followed by 91 percent of continuing costs. During its deliberations, however, the SFC considered expanding Medicaid along similar lines to the existing cost-sharing arrangement between the federal and state governments. Such a prospect provoked deep anxiety among the nation's governors, and the National Governors Association urged Senator Baucus to adopt the House approach.[33] In the end, this view prevailed. The Senate bill, which proposed that Medicaid provide health coverage up to 133 percent of the federal poverty level with federal funds to pay all the costs for three years and 90 percent thereafter, actually alleviated the concerns of "state officials" who "generally objected to the new Medicaid eligibility mandates."[34] Still, the ACA stipulated that any state that did not expand its Medicaid program would lose all its existing Medicaid federal funding.

The Senate and House also diverged over how to set up the insurance exchanges and especially how to allocate responsibilities among different levels of government. The House bill proposed that a new federal agency, known as the Health Choices Administration, would run a unified federal-level exchange, though states that wished to offer extended packages could opt out. The Senate bill called for states to set up their own exchanges, with the federal role restricted to a fallback plan if a state did not or could not set up its own scheme, and no penalties for states that failed to do so.[35] In many ways both bills expected the exchanges to perform the same functions. Both reform plans aimed to "enhance value, lower administrative costs, and foster competition in the insurance market by creating a health insurance exchange to facilitate choice and promote competition for enrollees."[36] Furthermore, both were to offer packages arranged in tiers, and both had provisions for redistributing risk. According to Timothy Jost, there were potential advantages to both state-based and federal exchanges. State-level exchanges had the advantage of wherewithal of local insurance and regulatory environments. But, as Jost asserts, markets operate much more efficiently nationally.[37] These latter advantages and the stronger federal role made the House version more attractive for liberals. As Jost explains, "Most importantly, a national program promises uniform implementation of the exchange," meaning that "no state will be allowed to simply refuse to set up an exchange, and then have the federal government step in belatedly and try to clean up the mess."[38]

The House bill, in short, would have put in place a much more centralized arrangement with considerably less discretion left to the states in terms of how the insurance exchanges would work. Interestingly, it was also a better fit with candidate Obama's health care plan, in which he called for a "National Health Insurance Exchange through which small businesses and individuals without access to other public programs or employer-based coverage could enroll in a new public plan, like Medicare, or in a range of approved private plans."[39] The Senate's approach reflected the preferences of the National Governors Association and many state-based lobbying groups as well as centrist Democrats such as Ben Nelson (D-NE).[40] It also illustrated the more moderate voting pivot point needed to pass legislation in the Senate rather than in the House (that is, a 60 percent filibuster-proof mark rather than a 50 percent-plus-1 simple-majority mark).

Also controversial was the question of how to introduce federal regulation of so-called medical loss ratios (MLR), which measure the extent to which insurance premiums are spent on providing health care. Prior to the ACA, thirty-two states had some form of MLR regulatory framework in place, but it was an area "largely ignored and . . . unregulated by the federal government."[41] A leading figure in pushing for more federal intervention was Senator Jay Rockefeller (D-WV), who, in a letter to the chief executive officer of the insurer Cigna, complained about how "large for-profit health insurers appear to be squeezing out more profit for Wall Street investors by spending a lower percentage of premium dollars on patient care than other insurers." Rockefeller said that he would attempt to introduce measures on the Senate floor that would set a "minimum" MLR for insurers.[42] The House bill did include a provision that insurers spend 85 percent of premiums on care, but that requirement extended only until 2013. In the Senate, however, Rockefeller and other advocates, such as Senator Al Franken from Minnesota, did manage to insert a very late provision into the Senate bill requiring insurers in the small-group and individual markets to spend 80 percent of premiums on care, a figure that rose to 85 percent in the large-group market.

According to Howard Dean, former chair of the Democratic National Committee, who had criticized the Senate for excluding the public option, the MLR regulation was the "most important thing of all . . . it requires insurance companies not to take quite as much off the top of your premiums as they have in the past."[43] Rockefeller and Franken had in fact called for the MLR to be set at 90 percent, but the Congressional Budget Office (CBO) said this would be too great a restriction on insurers' flexibility, and "in CBO's view, this further expansion of the federal government's role in the health insurance market would make such insurance an essentially government program," which effectively killed off that proposal.[44]

Although the inclusion of federal regulation of MLRs in the Senate bill was a defeat for the insurance industry, the language contained in the bill was not definitive because it left room for discretion in implementation. Even those sympathetic to the goals of MLR regulation emphasized that future oversight would be critical. For example, Kevin Lembo, head of the Office of the Healthcare Advocate in Connecticut, commented, "A lot goes back to the definition (of what is included in medical expenses), who is monitoring it, and how aggressively they do so."[45] Those details, however, were only to be filled in after legislation had been enacted, and the prospect of any law being passed hit an unexpected but potentially fatal roadblock in January 2010.

In 2009, when the Senate followed the House and passed a version of reform, the prevailing assumption was that although important differences between the

House and Senate bills needed to be ironed out in conference committee, the leading players in the process would find a way to the next step, and the president would be able to sign a health care reform bill.[46] That assumption, however, was blown away by the now famous "Massachusetts surprise," when Republican Scott Brown won a special election in that state to replace Senator Kennedy, who had died the previous summer. With no final bill agreed upon and the Democrats without their filibuster-proof majority in the Senate, it seemed as if the whole process had come to a shocking end. Furthermore, it seemed comprehensive health care reform would once again fall victim to the institutional fragmentation at the heart of US governance. This was particularly so because a central theme of Brown's campaign for the Senate was that he would provide the forty-first vote to block reform. When asked whether the reform effort was now finished, McConnell responded by saying, "I sure hope so."[47] Conservative commentator Fred Barnes declared, "It's safe to say no single Senate election in recent memory is as important as this one." He described how the result had weakened the president, would lead to panic among congressional Democrats, and spelled the end for health care reform.[48]

Barnes was proven wrong. After a period of uncertainty, the White House and its congressional allies decided that Speaker of the House Nancy Pelosi would attempt to recruit enough votes in the House to pass the Senate bill. This was not so straightforward a task because Pelosi needed to be able to assure her caucus that the Senate would then follow the House in passing a number of amendments to the original Senate bill. Afterward, the bill could be pushed through the Senate using the reconciliation process, thus circumventing a certain Republican filibuster.[49] The negotiations within Democratic ranks were fraught. According to former senator Tom Daschle, House Democrats thought the Senate bill was too compromised, to the extent that many "hated the Senate bill. *Despised* would not be too strong a word."[50] However, eventually there was agreement on a series of "fixes" to be included in the reconciliation bill, reaching a climax in the enactment of the ACA. The nature of the endgame, however, and the bypassing of a conference committee, had important consequences for the final policy design of the ACA, most particularly with regard to the organization of the health insurance exchanges.

In the short period between the passage of the Senate bill and the election of Brown, when attention prematurely turned to questions of how to reconcile the two versions of reform passed by the House and Senate respectively, an emerging area of debate was whether to follow the House plan for a national exchange or the Senate proposal of state-level exchanges. In support of the Senate bill, Senator Nelson said, "The national exchange is unnecessary, and I wouldn't support something that would start us down the road of federal regulation of insurance and a single-payer plan."[51] However, leading House Democrats were determined to fight for a national exchange, and it was by no means certain that the Senate version would have prevailed had the two versions of reform gone to conference committee.[52] Journalist E. J. Dionne reported that a deal was emerging that would bring the creation of a "national insurance exchange—alongside state exchanges," with the House "demanding this as the price for giving up on the public plan."[53] In the end, the result in Massachusetts brought this debate to a close. The rules of the reconciliation process could not be stretched to include fixing the Senate's version of the exchanges, locking state-based exchanges in place.[54]

In March 2010, with the Obama administration so relieved reform had been enacted, there was little expectation of how consequential the decision about whether to pursue state exchanges or a national one would be. At that time, the president and congressional leaders "assumed that every state would set up its own exchange."[55] Jacobs and Skocpol expected some state governments whose leaders were "unalterably opposed" to the ACA to choose not to set up an exchange but still predicted, "Most states will likely implement their own health exchanges, as Congress assumed."[56] There were, however, some cautionary voices. In early 2010, Jost noted how the ACA provided only limited funding to help states with the initial costs of setting up exchanges, meaning that in the long term the "exchange responsibilities are an unfunded mandate"; he further warned that previous efforts at "state-level implementation of federal health care reforms . . . have often been discouraging."[57]

It is impossible to second-guess what a national-level exchange would have looked like. The point here is not to argue that a federal exchange would have eliminated political opposition to the ACA's implementation. Instead, what becomes clear is that delegating the responsibility to the states, at least until the states forfeited that responsibility, provided institutional leverage for internal political actors to negotiate the terms under which they would set up the exchanges or more explicitly refuse to cooperate in dissent.

OPPOSING REFORM

As the ACA was being designed and enacted, the level of opposition to health care reform intensified and, significantly, was sustained after enactment throughout the implementation process. Some of the usual suspects, who had helped block reform efforts in the past, were in fact less vociferous than they had been previously because the White House had quickly decided to engage and compromise with the American Medical Association (AMA), the American Hospital Association (AHA), and the pharmaceutical industry.[58] Other actors and groups, however, refused to be pacified. Republicans in Washington, DC, and, perhaps even more

Table 2.1 Core Goals of Three Main Opponents before and after ACA Enactment

	Small Businesses	Insurance Industry	Republicans and Ideological Conservatives
Core goal during ACA enactment	Remove "individual mandate" and mandate on employers to insure their workers *Outcome: failed*	Remove the "public option" *Outcome: succeeded*	Prevent the enactment of the ACA altogether *Outcome: failed*
Core goal after ACA enactment	Reduce negative impact of ACA on employers; eliminate individual mandate	Make new regulations as favorable as possible to their perceived economic interests	Repeal and replace reform

importantly in the states mobilized in opposition to the ACA both before and after its enactment. Ideologically conservative groups kept up a drumbeat of hostility, and business groups and insurers lobbied to diminish the impact of aspects of the ACA they deemed damaging to their interests. Thus, although opponents failed to prevent the ACA from being enacted in the first place, they developed strategies aimed both at undermining public confidence in the efficacy of the law and more practically at obstructing or impairing implementation. Table 2.1 illustrates the main objectives of some ACA opponents.

Partisan and Ideological Opposition during Enactment

Unsurprisingly, the most public face of the opposition to Obamacare came from Republicans and conservative groups. Though Republicans and conservatives had sought ways to move toward universal health care, notably under President Richard Nixon, the Obama administration learned its lessons from the Clinton experience. Similarly, the GOP learned that opposing an ambitious attempt at policy reform and denouncing that plan as an attempt at a big-government takeover was a profitable political enterprise. In December 1993, a leading conservative strategist, Bill Kristol, distributed a memo to congressional Republicans urging them to "kill" Clinton's plan. Kristol's rationale was clearly laid out: if health care reform was successfully introduced, it "will revive the reputation of the party that spends and regulates, the Democrats, as the generous protector of middle-class interests. And it will at the same time strike a punishing blow against Republican claims to defend the middle class by restraining government."[59] In classic political science terms this could be seen as recognition of the idea that policy can remake politics.[60] That is, if people came to expect and actively access the benefits and services established by health care reform, then they would become protective of those benefits and reward the party that had put them in place.

Denouncing the reform effort as a big-government takeover paid political dividends. When President Clinton addressed a joint session of Congress in September 1993, the immediate reaction was positive.[61] Paul Starr, a key figure in designing the Clinton plan, later commented on the optimism generated by the media coverage of the speech: "At first it seemed Clinton would move the country. The next morning, Stanley Greenberg, the president's pollster, crowed that the overnight surveys showed we were winning two-thirds approval."[62] A year later the mood music was very different. The president was criticized for presenting a plan out of tune with American values. In the wake of the 1994 midterm elections, the reform effort was deemed to have caused significant political damage. Greenberg's crowing was replaced by a lament that the "health care defeat was catastrophic for Democrats."[63] By contrast, in 2010 the Republicans lost the battle in Congress but followed a similar playbook in terms of denouncing the ACA as the road to economic and moral ruin.

The attacks on the ACA as another big-government maneuver came despite the fact that the law was many steps away from resembling a Canadian-style single-payer system. The law's architects even claimed that some of its central ideas were borrowed from conservative sources. For example, the idea of the individual mandate had been previously touted by leading conservative think tank the Heritage Foundation, which had acknowledged in the early 1990s that any properly functioning insurance system required healthy individuals to buy insurance in order to avoid the problem of adverse selection.[64] However, Heritage Foundation members strenuously denied that the ideas that they had put forward sixteen years earlier were a prototype for Obamacare.[65]

Thus, forthright Republican opposition quickly became the party's default position, with GOP congressional leaders sometimes blaming Democrats for their lack of willingness to compromise. In an interview with Fox News host Greta Van Susteren in the wake of Brown's Senate victory in January 2010, House Minority Leader John Boehner said his Republican colleagues had consistently been willing to work with the president but had been "shut out, shut out, and shut out."[66] Acknowledging that GOP opposition had more strategic considerations, shortly before final passage of the ACA, McConnell explained how he had urged his caucus to remain steadfast in its opposition: "It was absolutely critical that everybody be together because if the proponents of the bill were able to say it was bipartisan, it tended to convey to the public that this is O.K. . . . It's either bipartisan or it isn't."[67] As the New York Times reported, McConnell's strategy of maintaining fierce public opposition to the developing legislation throughout 2009 could not stop the Senate from passing a bill, but it did pay some dividends by casting a shadow over the legitimacy of the Democratic achievement. "By the time the health bill was approved by the Senate on Christmas Eve with zero Republican votes, Democrats had been forced to cut questionable intraparty deals and jump through legislative hoops in an ugly process that helped sour the public on the party and its legislation."[68] As Patashnik and Zelizer explain, "Divisive enactment may undermine the credibility of the government's promise to stick with the new policy, which discourages the organizational adaptations needed to make the policy effective."[69] So the Democrats had their "prize," but it was a tarnished one, leaving opponents to claim they were justified in continuing active efforts to thwart the law's intent.[70]

One feature of the reform debate throughout 2009 was the manner in which Republican lawmakers came under growing pressure from conservative ideological groups. The partisan interests of the Republicans and the policy preferences of conservative groups generally converged through the legislative process, but when it appeared as if the unity of opposition Senator McConnell championed might crack, outside groups were determined to enforce an ideological purity.[71] In this context, as opposition to health care reform fueled the rise of the Tea Party in summer 2009, the congressional recess brought town hall meetings disrupted by antireform protestors, though pro- and antireform advocates disagreed about whether these protests were organic or artificially manufactured by wealthy backers. These disruptions mobilized activists around the theme of antistatism, which, in turn, reinforced the absolutist nature of Republican opposition on Capitol Hill.[72] More directly, the Club for Growth, a prominent supporter of conservative causes known to back primary challenges against insufficiently conservative Republican legislators, announced that it would begin to run advertisements in the home states of the three Republicans in the SFC's Gang of Six urging them not to make any concessions to Democratic plans. The head of the Club for Growth Chris Chocola, a former US representative from Indiana, noted, "We believe it is vital that these three Republican senators do not cave in to the far left."[73] Despite Senator Snowe's vote in favor of reporting the bill out of SFC, another Republican member of the Gang of Six, Senator Grassley, denounced the SFC's bill as setting down a "slippery slope toward more and more government control of health care."[74]

Interest-Group Opposition during Enactment

Employers have long been the primary providers of health insurance in the United States, and the ACA did not propose to challenge this arrangement. However, although large employers who already provided insurance to workers were concerned by the rising costs of providing that benefit, smaller employers were much more concerned about the parts of the ACA that mandated employers with more than fifty workers to provide insurance. In 1993 and 1994, small business opposition, organized into the National Federation of Independent Business (NFIB), combined very effectively with small health insurers, who were then represented by the Health Insurers Association of America (HIAA) to campaign against the Clinton reform. The NFIB used intensive lobbying to oppose an employer mandate even before the details of the Health Security Act were revealed, and the HIAA funded the famous (or notorious) Harry and Louise advertisements.[75] Sixteen years later the NFIB remained a powerful voice against any reform, including an employer mandate, and the American Association of Health Insurance Providers (AHIP) was more circumspect than its predecessor, HIAA, had been. AHIP in fact made overtures to the Obama campaign in summer 2008 to indicate that AHIP would trade a mandate on its members to accept anyone who applied for insurance in return for a requirement that everyone purchase insurance.[76] Nevertheless, the White House and insurers were only ever uneasy allies at best, and the latter vociferously opposed the idea of a public option and were wary of rules governing MLRs and restrictions on insurer practices.

Postenactment Opposition Strategies

Republican partisans and conservative groups did little to change their tune even after the ACA became the law of the land, calling for the law's repeal. For Republican legislators, this demand had electoral appeal, and for conservative groups it represented their determination to limit the role of the state in health care provision.[77] In reality, repeal in Washington was beyond the immediate institutional capacity of the ACA's opponents, but other effective avenues for challenging the law remained. The first strategy was to obstruct implementation as much as possible by exploiting the fact that much of that implementation was to be done at the state level, where ACA opponents remained powerful players.[78] Second, they would maintain a vigorous critique of the ACA and use the issue to mobilize activists with an eye to the 2010 elections. Success in those elections, at the state level as well as at the congressional level, would further reinforce their capacity to obstruct implementation, particularly because the vast bulk of the ACA's rules and regulations were to come into force only after these midterm elections. As Figure 2.1 shows, the timeline for ACA implementation was gradual, with state governments central to that process. Third, they would challenge the ACA in the courts. These challenges might be successful, and the very fact that the law was being dragged through the courts would add to a sense of public unease about its legitimacy.

From spring 2010 onward, conservatives waged a very public campaign denouncing the law as wasteful and bad for the economy, which "legitimized" their

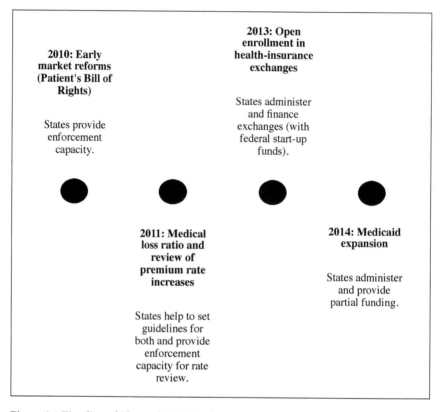

2010: Early market reforms (Patient's Bill of Rights)

States provide enforcement capacity.

2013: Open enrollment in health-insurance exchanges

States administer and finance exchanges (with federal start-up funds).

2011: Medical loss ratio and review of premium rate increases

States help to set guidelines for both and provide enforcement capacity for rate review.

2014: Medicaid expansion

States administer and provide partial funding.

Figure 2.1 Timeline of Planned ACA Implementation

Note: Includes only major reforms covered in this book. For a more encompassing list of changes, please see citation.

Source: US Department of Health and Human Services, "Key Features of the Affordable Care Act by Year," accessed December 1, 2014, http://www.hhs.gov/healthcare/facts/timeline/timeline-text .html#2010.

strategy of obstructing implementation. The fact that so much implementation was delegated to the states meant another legislative battleground opened up, or perhaps more accurately, fifty new battlegrounds opened up after Washington had finished its work. Prior to the 1990s, the emphasis in debates about national health care reform was placed on the *national,* with the states' "subordinate role . . . taken for granted."[79] Following the collapse of the Clinton reform effort, there was renewed debate about the appropriate role of the states, though some states acted more aggressively to expand access to insurance and/or regulate insurers than others did. Although rates of uninsured per state did not provide a straightforward barometer of public policy effort, the disparities in the year before Obama became president were stark. In 2008, eight states plus the District of Columbia had rates of uninsured lower than 10 percent. Massachusetts, where 5 percent of the population was uninsured, had the lowest rate. At the other end of the scale, six states had rates of uninsured above 19 percent, with Texas topping the list with the number of uninsured at 24.5 percent.[80] For liberal Democrats, this divergence revealed the importance of imposing national standards with as much federal control as possible. In the end, however, as Figure 2.1 illustrates, the design of reform meant that state governments were going to have to act as honest brokers rather than bystanders to be bypassed if the promises made by reform advocates were to be delivered.

Importantly, the capacity of dissidents to obstruct the reform varied from one aspect of policy to another according to the design of the ACA and the institutional leverage it afforded opponents across the different provisions of the law. As the ACA was written, states had wide discretion in the establishment of the insurance exchange marketplaces. State-level actors would be key in negotiating with insurers over the MLR and insurance premium regulations, especially because much of the law remained vague, with details to be decided by administrative agencies.[81] In contrast, the Medicaid expansion initially appeared to be a policy area in which a national standard had effectively been put in place. Although states were in quite different starting positions in terms of developing the bureaucratic capacity to implement the expansion, the prohibitive sanctions proposed for states not participating in the expansion did mean that there seemed to be little room for dissent.

Opponents' efforts to sabotage implementation and to organize dissent at the state level began immediately, with the American Legislative Exchange Council (ALEC) leading the way. ALEC urged state lawmakers to adopt, either as law or as a constitutional amendment, the "Freedom of Choice in Health Care Act," a piece of model legislation the group had drawn up. Doing this, ALEC claimed, would "provide a state-level defense against Obamacare's excessive federal power."[82] On March 10, 2010, Virginia became the first state to adopt a law closely following the ALEC model, and Idaho quickly followed suit. A plethora of measures was introduced in other state legislatures to rebuke the ACA or, more practically, demand that state agencies not take action to implement various aspects of the law.[83]

The likelihood of cooperation versus resistance to ACA implementation clearly depended on the makeup of state governments, meaning the law's opponents put huge energy into the 2010 elections. These elections, pivotal to the future implementation of the ACA, brought thirty-seven contests for gubernatorial mansions, with the Democrats defending nineteen and the GOP eighteen. An indication of the intensity of competition can be seen in the levels of campaign contributions to statewide races, which exceeded both 2008 and 2012 levels. Figure 2.2 shows that contributions to statewide races, including governors, legislatures, state courts, and

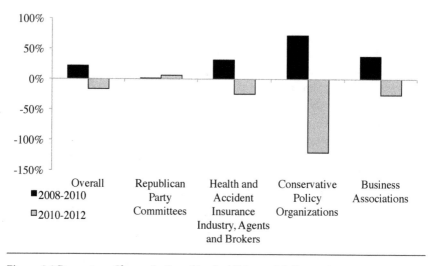

Figure 2.2 Percentage Change in Spending in All Statewide Races, 2008–2012
Source: Calculated by the authors using followthemoney.org.

other elected offices, increased 21.47 percent between 2008 and 2010 and declined 16.20 percent between 2010 and 2012. Contributions by insurers and brokers increased 31.59 percent between 2008 and 2010 and fell by more than 24 percent thereafter. Business associations displayed a magnified version of this pattern. Yet the most dramatic increase in spending was among conservative policy organizations in the states, whose contributions to statewide races increased by more than 70 percent between 2008 and 2010 and fell 120.66 percent between 2010 and 2012.

From a conservative perspective this was money well spent. Building on a wave of conservative populism, partisan turnover in the states in favor of Republicans was especially robust. As Table 2.2 shows, the number of Republican governors increased in the 2010 elections from twenty-three to twenty-nine governors, and the number of seats in state legislatures held by Republicans increased from 3,282 to 3,890. This was a landslide of historic proportions, meaning there were "now more Republican state legislators than [at] any time since the Great Depression."[84] Most importantly, this meant the number of states with unified Republican government (two solid Republican chambers and a Republican governor) increased from eight to eighteen states. This allowed opponents of the ACA in Republican-dominated states to rely on state officials as potential veto points for the reform. Where legislatures were not involved in the reform, Republican-appointed insurance commissioners, attorneys general, and Medicaid directors could issue other sorts of challenges—either in the regulatory process or in implementation of the law itself.

Table 2.2 Shifts in Partisan Control of State Government, 2008–2010

	Before 2010 Elections	After 2010 Elections	Percentage Shift
Number and percentage of states with Republican governor	23 (46%)	29 (58%)	+12%
Number and percentage of Republican seats in state legislatures	3,282 (44.5%)	3,890 (52.7%)	+8%
Number and percentage of states with unified Republican control of state government	8 (16%)	18 (36%)	+20%

Source: Compiled by authors from Ballotpedia.com.

These victories at the state level were also matched in Washington, DC, where the GOP took control of the House, with anti-"Obamacare" backlash propelling the Republican wave.[85] This did not give Republicans sufficient leverage for repeal, but it gave them a platform for rhetorical opposition and ruled out the possibility of amendments friendly to the ACA to deal with any emerging problems relatively easily corrected by legislative action. House Republicans were simply not interested in remedying the law, arguing mostly that flaws embedded in the 2010 law disrupted the rollout of health care reform.[86]

The third opposition strategy was to challenge the ACA in the courts. In its own way, the ACA acted as a miniature stimulus bill for the legal industry, with opponents quickly taking up various challenges to the law. In itself, the opponents' decision to turn to the courts was unsurprising, though the nature of the challenges and the willingness of some courts to accommodate the challenges were much less predictable. The most high-profile dispute concerned the constitutionality of the individual mandate. Led by Florida, twenty-six states and allied business groups combined forces, asserting that compelling people to buy health insurance was an attempt to regulate economic inactivity, which fell outside of the established power of Congress to regulate actual existing economic activity. In June 2012, in the case of the *National Federation of Independent Business (NFIB) v. Sebelius,* the Supreme Court ruled the mandate constitutional by a five-to-four majority.[87] The administration's relief, however, was undercut by the manner in which the Court gave more consideration than anticipated to a further challenge to the ACA regarding the Medicaid expansion.[88]

Although it upheld the essential constitutionality of the ACA, the Supreme Court's intervention with regard to the law's Medicaid provisions was significant, effectively rewriting the policy design behind the proposed expansion. As originally set out, the ACA intended to ensure that all states participated in the expansion, but by a seven-to-two majority the Court ruled that the condition that states conform or lose their existing Medicaid funding from the federal government constituted unacceptable levels of fiscal bullying.[89] In short, the Court determined that the ACA did not in reality give the states any choice about whether to participate because the cost of nonparticipation was unreasonable. This ruling meant that, although the fiscal incentive to participate endured because the carrot of potentially significant federal funds for each state remained in play, the stick, which to all intents and purposes would have made participation compulsory, was taken away. Reflecting on the Court's decision, James Morone commented that in its original form the ACA had "very quietly . . . introduced a revolutionary change: All poor people in America would get Medicaid." The Court's decision, however, meant that "stingy states may choose to stay stingy."[90]

The Court had created the opportunity for state actors to dissent from the terms of the ACA. One leading governor, Rick Perry in Texas, promptly declared his state would not expand its Medicaid program even though Texas had the highest rate of uninsured in the nation.[91] In addition, the Court's decision changed the dynamics of the relationship between federal and state authorities in more subtle ways. The Medicaid expansion had effectively been an instruction from the federal government to the states to fulfill one of the core ambitions of health care reformers. By taking away the capacity of the federal government to instruct in this manner, the Court handed states new institutional leverage and bargaining power with the federal government to explore alternative means of achieving the goals intended by the Medicaid expansion.

The Medicaid rebuff was not the only defeat for the ACA in the Supreme Court. At the end of June 2014, the Court, by a five-to-four majority, ruled against the Obama administration in *Burwell v. Hobby Lobby Stores, Inc.* In this case, the Court ruled that employers could not be compelled to include certain types of contraception as part of the insurance they offered to their employees if this offended their religious beliefs.[92] Although this case raises interesting ethical questions, it does not directly affect the questions about intergovernmental relations addressed in this book, except to the extent that it further fueled public skepticism about the efficacy of the law, and it certainly gave opponents a further chance to allege the ACA as an example of big-government overreach that should be resisted. For example, Grace-Marie Turner of the conservative Galen Institute commented, "The government's loss ignites a fresh challenge to the Obama administration's often-illegal implementation of the health overhaul law."[93]

A more fundamental legal challenge also came to the fore in July 2014 when the District of Columbia Court of Appeals, by a two-to-one margin, supported a case that would fatally undermine the way in which the federally organized state exchanges were working. This case, brought in *Halbig v. Burwell,* revolved around the idea that federal subsidies granted through insurance exchanges to households up to 400 percent of the FPL could be given only when the exchanges were set up and run by the state. The decision primarily hinged on the language used in the ACA. All sides agreed that section 1311 "provides that states 'shall' establish exchanges, but since Congress cannot literally require states to do so, section 1321 provides that if a state 'elects' not to establish the 'required' exchange, the Department of Health and Human Services shall establish 'such' exchange for the state."[94] The disagreement was over whether a federally facilitated exchange was in fact an exchange established by the state because section 36B, which explains the availability of subsidies, refers to exchanges created in section 1311 (that is, an exchange created by the state, not the federal government). In its interpretation of the law, the Internal Revenue Service (IRS), as the federal agency responsible for determining eligibility for subsidies through the exchanges, decided that the intent of the ACA was clearly for all exchanges to be treated equally in terms of the subsidies. The DC Circuit Court, however, found that the language in section 36B did specifically preclude subsidies being granted through the federally facilitated exchanges.[95] Hence, according to this ruling the IRS had overstepped its authority, and subsidies should not be granted to people accessing insurance through the federally run exchanges. Prior to the District of Columbia Court ruling, lower courts had sided with the administration, agreeing that subsidies could also be granted through the federally run exchanges. In fact on the same day as the *Halbig* ruling, the US Court of Appeals for the Fourth Circuit decided *King v. Burwell.* The case covered the same ground, but this court issued a different judgment. This time, the judges ruled that although the language of the ACA was certainly ambiguous, the law's intent to maximize access to insurance was not, and the IRS's interpretation should therefore stand.[96] In November 2014 the Supreme Court decided to intervene by hearing an appeal in the *King* case. In June 2015, this challenge to the ACA was defeated when the Supreme Court, by a six-to-three majority, decided the case in the administration's favor. However, reflecting the pressured environment in which the legislative process had been brought to a conclusion, Chief Justice Roberts expressed his view that the ACA contained "more than a few examples of inartful drafting" that did "not reflect the type of care and deliberation that one might expect of such significant legislation."[97]

Legal questions aside, the *King* and *Halbig* cases provide important insight into the nature of the opposition to the ACA. These challenges to the law did not spring organically from aggrieved individuals but reflected organized action by steadfast opponents in the wake of the Supreme Court's decision in *NFIB v. Sebelius.* The *Washington Post* reported on the *Halbig* case: "Conservatives have spent years laying the groundwork for the challenge, which they considered their last, best chance at hollowing out the federal program. Activists had lobbied state legislatures, urging them not to set up their own marketplaces in part to magnify the effect if the courts ruled their way."[98] In turn this illustrates how the three strategies of obstructing implementation, winning political power in the states, and taking the ACA to the courts combined to sustain the effectiveness of opposition to the health care reform well after the law's passage in spring 2010.

CONCLUSION

What emerges from this chapter is a complex story of an uncertain legislative victory. The passage of the ACA was a major legislative achievement for the Obama administration and the congressional Democratic leadership. The president and his congressional allies succeeded where others had failed. Yet, much of the story has been about the compromises made along the way, leaving some analysts sympathetic to the aims of reform to lament that the ACA was a "muddle-through bill," determined by the need of lawmakers on the margin of any reform-minded coalition to win votes.[99] However, the compromises did not mollify opponents and, even as it was being developed, the ACA was sowing some of the seeds that came to haunt it when the major elements of the implementation process began.

In choosing to build on the employer-based system of health insurance and delegating significant parts of implementation of the law to the states, the ACA allowed plenty of scope for private interests and political opponents to contest and undermine the law's objectives. As we will see over the next chapters, those interests did not always ally with the political opponents, and in fact those partisan opponents at the state level were sometimes more cooperative than their rhetoric suggested. Still, reformers never established their control over the postenactment turf in a decisive fashion.

As we will show, it is wrong to overgeneralize about the fate of the ACA. Some aspects proved more susceptible to cooperative engagement between federal and state actors than others. Moreover, the fiscal and institutional incentives across the three areas we study in depth were different, as was the level of public understanding and scrutiny. Hence, the state-level battles over health care reform implementation played out in strikingly divergent ways across the law's major provisions.

3. Health Insurance Exchanges: When Dissent Means "Not Lifting a Finger"[1]

Relatively uncontroversial during the enactment of the Patient Protection and Affordable Care Act (ACA), health insurance exchanges (also known as health insurance marketplaces) rapidly became one of the most contested aspects of the federal health reform in the states, especially those controlled by the Republicans. In Florida, for example, Governor Rick Scott not only rejected the idea of state-run exchanges central to the ACA but also launched an outright political battle in 2013 against the federal government over issues such as the "security of people's personal information as they sign up for health coverage under the Affordable Care Act."[1] In a context of exacerbated partisanship, states such as Florida had to choose between constructing new institutions from scratch and declining to do so. Because many Republican-controlled states chose the latter course, implementing a seemingly promarket policy instrument such as the health insurance exchange proved much less cooperative terrain than anticipated. Yet, although partisan opposition to the ACA goes a long way toward explaining why many states governed by Republicans dissented in the case of the exchanges, as the following chapters will show, partisan opposition is not enough to explain why dissent was such a prominent part of postreform politics in the case of exchanges but less so in the cases of Medicaid and regulatory reform. Rather, the evidence here suggests that the absence of strong policy legacy, strong institutional fragmentation, and mixed public sentiments toward the individual mandate and the ACA as a whole made it particularly easy for partisan opponents of the reform to dissent from exchange provisions.

To a greater degree than with Medicaid expansion, which came with significant federal fiscal incentives, health insurance exchanges became the object of a highly symbolic conservative mobilization against the ACA as the conservative push to reject state-run exchanges paved the road to the multiplication of federally led exchanges in many red states. In other words, the conservative crusade against state-run exchanges increased the role of the federal government and, consequently, of the Department of Health and Human Services (HHS) and Barack Obama's administration in ACA implementation.

This chapter begins by detailing the history and institutional features of health insurance exchanges as they developed during and after the enactment of the ACA. We follow this discussion with an analysis of patterns of consent in the states and feature the case of California, the first state that agreed to create its own exchange. This analysis leads to a longer section on the politics of dissent in the states that culminates in the presentation of our additional cases: an example of strong dissent (Texas) and three hybrid cases that featured mixed patterns of dissent and consent (North Carolina, Arkansas, and Missouri).

ESTABLISHING HEALTH INSURANCE MARKETPLACES: THE POLICY ISSUES

Under the ACA, exchanges are meant to help "uninsured people find health coverage,"[2] notably through the selection and regulation of affordable health insurance plans and the identification of citizens eligible for federal subsidies, that is, those with incomes less than 400 percent of the poverty level. More generally, as William Brandon and Keith Carnes suggest, "Exchanges describe and facilitate the sale of complicated products in a regulated manner intended to minimize the information asymmetry that often exists between buyers and sellers of complex goods such as health insurance."[3] In this context, the extension of the exchange model to health care appears to be a logical step, at least from the perspective of a market-friendly approach such as the one embedded in the ACA. Yet, according to Brandon and Carnes, the analogy between stock exchanges and health insurance exchanges is potentially misleading; whereas the latter must become "fully transparent and accessible to ordinary individuals," this is not necessarily the case of the former.[4] This is why access to basic information about health insurance is such a central issue in the ongoing debate about the design and implementation of health insurance exchanges in the United States. From this perspective, access to "navigators" tasked to guide ordinary citizens through the complex world of health insurance is crucial.[5] At the same time, designing easy-to-use websites people can access without prior knowledge or training is essential from both policy and political standpoints. This is true because the exchange website becomes the public face of the exchange and, indirectly, the public face of the ACA. In this context, in late summer and early fall 2013, the problems with the federal exchange website became so toxic for the Obama administration not only because they jeopardized exchange-based enrollment but also because websites are among the most visible aspects of the ACA, through which many citizens are meant to discover the potential benefits granted to them. This is why health insurance exchanges are destined to provide the "democratic consumer experience of buying an airline seat through Expedia

.com or Travelocity."[6] Although health insurance exchanges have a much broader mission than these online booking sites, the analogy is useful because it draws our attention to the fundamental role of their information technology component.

More specifically, in the context of the ACA, health insurance exchanges are meant to fulfill a number of core tasks that have become embroiled in political controversy. First, exchanges played a significant role in the attempt to increase the number of Americans with access to affordable insurance coverage.[7] This, however, became highly contentious because it was associated with the "individual mandate." Although the exchanges were not explicitly tied to the mandate in the ACA because the vast majority of people would be insured through means other than an exchange, there was some institutional overlap between the management of subsidies through the exchanges and the enforcement of the individual mandate because the Internal Revenue Service (IRS) was charged with a key role in the administration of these actions.[8] Hence, state decisions about setting up exchanges have become politically salient, especially for people purchasing insurance on the exchanges.

Second, creating an exchange means establishing benchmark plans under the ACA's essential health benefits provisions, which define minimum categories of coverage.[9] Such provisions seek to improve market coverage by ensuring that people cannot purchase low-quality, inadequate health insurance. Importantly, these ACA provisions define "essential health benefits" only in broad terms, thus leaving much power to HHS and the states to define the precise content of adequate insurance coverage during the implementation process. Issues related to quality standards directly affect the health insurance coverage citizens and consumers are likely to receive.[10]

Finally, regarding the administration of exchanges, the ACA specifies partial preemption of state law. If states refuse to create exchanges, HHS is obligated to establish them to serve these states. States can operate exchanges only if they meet minimum operating standards; doing this requires states to facilitate technical transfer and manage risk, among other tasks.[11] Taking responsibility for planning and management is a critical political issue because the identity of the level of government effectively controlling exchanges and their implementation is likely to shape the allocation of credit for positive policy outcomes and blame for negative outcomes.[12]

POLICY LEGACIES, INSTITUTIONAL FRAGMENTATION, AND PUBLIC SENTIMENTS

The idea of health insurance exchanges for both uninsured individuals and small businesses took shape in the early 1990s and thus predated the popularization of the Internet; as Alain Enthoven shows, this directly influenced the content of President Clinton's ill-fated Health Security Act.[13] Centered on the concept of "managed competition,"[14] however, President Clinton's Health Insurance Purchasing Cooperatives (later called Health Alliances) differed considerably from the health insurance exchanges created as part of the ACA. For example, Clinton's approach "relied principally on an employer mandate to purchase insurance for workers, whereas Obama relies on an individual mandate."[15] More importantly, health insurance exchanges as part of the ACA are more modest in scope than the Health Alliances of the Health Security Act; they only target small businesses and uninsured individuals instead of becoming the only source of market-based health insurance coverage. Consequently, although their role is essential within the ACA, contemporary health insurance exchanges are residual in nature because their core mission is simply to complement existing forms of health insurance provision.[16]

As a consensual and market-friendly idea, the health insurance exchanges initially proved relatively uncontroversial and even popular among some Republican policy makers because they were closely associated with the Massachusetts bipartisan health insurance reform enacted in 2006 during the governorship of future Republican presidential candidate Mitt Romney. Prior to and during the enactment of the ACA, exchanges had been a bipartisan idea, but aside from "Romneycare," they were *only* an idea. Though all states had some authority to regulate health insurance markets prior to the ACA, virtually none had the power to create a marketplace for the sale and purchase of health plans. The absence of this preexisting legacy would become important as Republican policy makers turned against health insurance exchanges *after* the ACA's enactment. This new opposition had little to do with the nature of this market-friendly policy instrument, which features a subsidization of private health coverage that, to a certain extent, makes the ACA a "voucher bill."[17] Rather, as David Jones, Katherine Bradley, and Jonathan Oberlander put it, in the hyperpartisan, post-ACA world, "Exchanges became controversial largely because they suffered from guilt by association—with Democrats, President Obama, and Obamacare."[18] Because virtually no states had exchanges "up and running," they were ripe ground for partisan and ideological contestation.

Adding to the thin policy legacies of the exchanges, the ACA's fragmented design created a unique window of opportunity for conservative, Republican opponents in the states to engage in dissent. The central role of the states in exchange implementation is the result of a political decision made during the enactment process. The House version of the bill did not give the states the capacity to implement health insurance exchanges whatsoever. According to the House bill, "The federal government would have been solely responsible for operating exchanges."[19] However, the Senate rejected this approach; instead, state insurance commissioners, governors, and centrist Democrats wielded more influence in drafting the bill and prevailed upon senators to rely on state officials' experience and expertise by giving them the option of running the exchanges.[20] In the end, after the victory of Scott Brown in the January 2010 Massachusetts Senate race, the more decentralized vision of the health insurance exchanges embedded in the Senate's version became law, and the House bill featuring a purely federal exchange was discarded altogether.

Yet Congress did more than decentralize administrative authority. In expecting states to establish institutions that had never before existed at the state level and would eventually be self-financing, it necessitated action on the part of governors and legislatures to change the status quo. Administrative agencies could not simply create exchanges on their own. This made exchanges a perfect target for opponents of the law because challenging them did not actually require building legislative coalitions. Rather, opponents could engage in dissent by stalling the passage of legislation establishing an exchange, which, given the many veto points in the legislative process, was especially easy.

To be sure, Congress incentivized the creation of exchanges through providing $4.8 billion in grants to the states and a more modest federal "fallback" should states refuse.[21] Yet these incentives alone did not change the fact that few state governments had preexisting authority to establish insurance exchanges. Because exchanges were styled as a policy innovation, state agencies and governors could not quietly take federal money while bargaining over the terms of reform. Although the governors of two states—Kentucky and New York—established exchanges through executive orders, the battle would have to be fought in state legislative chambers—treacherous territory for Obamacare.

Moreover, Congress provided no clear punishments for states that did not create their own exchanges. Though conservative litigants argued later that Congress did not intend for the IRS to provide premium tax-credit subsidies to states that opted out of creating an exchange, they did so only after the *National Federation of Independent Business (NFIB) v. Sebelius* Supreme Court decision of June 2012, and virtually no state officials that refused the exchanges saw themselves as sacrificing premium tax credits.[22] Public statements by Republican governors and legislatures, policy evaluations by state planning committees, and comments submitted by state agencies pursuant to the release of the IRS final rule on tax credits complained of federal controls on state exchanges and federal spending on intergovernmental grants but made no mention of premium tax credits.[23] As Governor Dave Heineman (R-NE) put it in November 2012, Nebraska refused to create the exchange because of its high cost but admitted that "on the key issues . . . there is no real operational difference between a federal exchange and a state exchange."[24] After the *NFIB v. Sebelius* decision, only Oklahoma added the tax-credit issue to its pending federal lawsuits, and, even then, the state advised eligible citizens that they "qualify for the federal Health Insurance Marketplace and related advance premium tax credits."[25]

Finally, although the idea of exchanges remained popular among most *voters,* with favorability polling at or above 80 percent between 2010 and 2013, exchanges were perceived as being linked to the new mechanism by which the public would experience the law's *least* popular (and most salient) provision: the individual mandate. By way of comparison, public support for the mandate never rose *above* 40 percent during the first four years of implementation. Republican governors and state legislators could easily convert the exchanges into a flashpoint of opposition to "Obamacare." Without fearing popular reprisal, they could engage in combat more real than symbolic, turning back millions of dollars in federal grant money and sending uninsured residents to federally run marketplaces.

Overall, a combination of thin policy legacies, institutional fragmentation, and mixed public sentiments in the fragmented context of US federalism helps explain the high level of conflict over the implementation of health insurance exchanges witnessed in a large number of states controlled at least in part by Republicans. This opposition proves particularly strong because, in terms of policy design and in contrast to the situation prevailing in the field of Medicaid expansion, states have limited financial incentives to implement their own exchanges because existing federal subsidies aim only at helping states set up such exchanges.

THE NEGOTIATION OF CONSENT

In this challenging institutional and political context, HHS hoped to foster consent and collaboration on the part of Republican-controlled states. Its strategy was to encourage as many states as possible to set up their own exchanges when issuing regulations about the health insurance exchanges.[26] In fact, immediately after the enactment of the ACA, the federal government began discussing rules regarding issues such as "minimum requirements" with states for plans that would become available through the exchanges. From the beginning, federal officials seemed willing to negotiate with their state counterparts to facilitate the implementation process. This is true because, at all stages of that process, "federal officials had a strong interest in persuading state officials to take on as many exchange tasks as possible."[27] HHS provided flexibility to the states and frequently agreed to negotiate with them over key implementation issues.[28]

After the 2010 midterm elections, with opposition to the ACA and state-operated exchanges in GOP-controlled states growing, HHS recognized new, hybrid forms of exchanges that allowed for diverse forms of state participation. For HHS, having as many states as possible participate in exchange implementation was especially important because setting up exchanges in many states proved expensive and created extra pressure on the federal government not anticipated during the legislative process, when exchanges proved uncontroversial. This meant most states were expected to prefer to create their own exchanges rather than leave Washington to take care of it. In a changing political and partisan context in which exchanges suffered from "guilt by association," HHS rapidly adapted to show a high level of policy flexibility, made possible by the fact that many of the details regarding the implementation of exchanges had not been included in the ACA. Such a policy design allowed federal bureaucrats to issue guidelines and regulations that made exchanges potentially more palatable to states reluctant to implement them on their own. For instance, in May 2012, "to provide a middle ground" between state and purely federal exchanges, the "federal government introduced a new option not included in the ACA: a federal-state partnership exchange."[29] According to this new policy design option, states would not directly create their own exchanges but would play a direct role in their operation through collaboration with the federal government, which adopted an increasingly pragmatic and open approach to accommodate the needs of more reluctant states and foster greater levels of collaboration. Later on, other hybrid models emerged, with the blessing of HHS, which afforded even more flexibility to reluctant states.[30]

Another form of flexibility introduced by HHS concerned the deadlines for states to announce whether they would create their own health insurance exchanges. After extending these deadlines several times, with the hope that more states would decide to participate at a later date, HHS finally declared that such deadlines no longer existed and that states could take over existing federal exchanges later, as long as they met existing federal requirements.[31] As journalist Robert Pear stated in the *New York Times*, "A political benefit of this strategy is that it allows the administration to keep working with even the most recalcitrant states. Administration officials said they were trying to persuade such states to share the work of running an exchange, supervising health plans, and assisting consumers."[32] The limits of this approach are outlined later in this chapter, in the section about the politics of dissent. For now, we turn to the politics of consent and how it materialized in the months following the adoption of the ACA.

A Soft Case for Consent: California as "Early Adopter"

Flexibility on the part of the federal government to facilitate consent and cooperation was not necessary in all parts of the country. Despite ongoing ideological and political controversy surrounding the ACA, there are clear examples of strong and unambiguous political consent. Unsurprisingly, such examples are typically found in more liberal states at least partially controlled by Democrats. Interestingly, the first state to enact legislation to create its own health insurance exchange system in the aftermath of the ACA featured a Republican governor, Arnold Schwarzenegger. A more liberal state in terms of public sentiments, where the majority of the population supported the ACA,[33] California nonetheless witnessed the mobilization of insurance companies and business organizations against the anticipated decision of Governor Schwarzenegger to proceed rapidly with the development of state-run health insurance exchanges.[34] On the one hand, insurance companies claimed that the strong bargaining power granted to the proposed California Health Benefits Exchange would crush their business and, thus, hurt consumers. For instance, Anthem Blue Cross asserted "that setting rates in the exchange would likely politicize the rate-setting process, which has proven to lead to insurer insolvency and insurers withdrawing from the market, reducing choices for consumers."[35] On the other hand, in a last-minute attempt to convince the governor not to sign two pieces of legislation (Assembly Bill 1602 and Senate Bill 900) authorizing the creation of the California Health Benefits Exchange, in late September 2010, the California Chamber of Commerce, the California Taxpayers' Association, and the National Federation of Independent Business/California published a full page ad in the *Los Angeles Times* attacking the proposed exchange model because of what they depicted as insufficient oversight:

> These two bills give five political appointees authority to run a new bureaucracy that will buy health insurance for millions of Californians, all with little guidance or oversight. When fully functional, the Exchange could have an annual budget of as much as $40 billion. Yet, the bills exempt Exchange employees from state civil service pay caps, allow the Exchange to set its rules with only limited public review, and let the Board conduct some meetings in secret.

Although these three organizations did not oppose the idea of state-sponsored exchanges, they warned the governor against signing these particular pieces of legislation:

> Your governorship has been marked by efforts to reform government, reduce burdensome taxes, and rid waste from the state's budget. We respectfully ask you to veto AB 1602 and SB 900. It is critical that we get health care reform right, and we stand ready to work with the Administration and Legislature to craft a proposal that will assure efficiency, protect taxpayers, and provide proper oversight and accountability to the public.[36]

However, less than a week after that ad appeared and barely six months after the adoption of the controversial ACA, Governor Schwarzenegger signed the two laws that set the course for the creation of the California Health Benefits Exchange.[37] This early decision to set up the California Health Benefits Exchange was particularly important because of the sheer size of the state, by far the most populous in the nation (more than 37 million people in 2010, higher than the population of Canada). Partly because of this, in 2010 a study estimated that approximately 4 million people would enroll in the California Health Benefits Exchange by 2016.[38] Considering the magnitude of the task at hand, establishing that exchange and implementing other aspects of the ACA in California represented a true policy challenge, especially in light of the negative fiscal situation of the state at the time. The state's fiscal problems in fact had less of an impact on decisions regarding the exchange than in the case of Medicaid expansion because, as discussed in the next chapter, the state's Medi-Cal program faced great fiscal pressures.[39]

In 2012, after much discussion and consultation about branding, the California Health Benefits Exchange became Covered California, a much shorter and user-friendly term.[40] The governance structure of this new public organization is straight-forward: "Covered California is an independent public entity with a five-member governing board of directors. The board's membership consists of the secretary of the California Department of Health and Human Services or the secretary's desig-nee and four other California residents—two appointed by the governor, one by the speaker of the Assembly, and one by the Senate Committee on Rules."[41] In a state where support for the ACA was higher than the national average, the creation of the state exchanges proved less controversial than in other regions of the country, which does not mean enrollment, which began in October 2013, proceeded without any glitches. For instance, the CoveredCA.com website faced minor problems, and "one insurer, Alameda Alliance, was dropped in November because it failed to get necessary state licensure to sell on the Exchange. This reduced number of insurers on the Exchange to 11."[42] By April 2014, the initial enrollment campaign produced higher-than-expected results in California. This is true because a "concerted, late-stage effort by California's health insurance exchange to expand outreach efforts, particularly in Latino communities, helped boost private health insurance sign-ups in the Golden State to almost 1.4 million."[43] Commenting on these enrollment numbers and those for the federally operated exchanges, University of California–Los Angeles (UCLA) health care policy professor Gerald Kominski even declared to the *San Jose Mercury News*, "It's a Super Bowl moment, and Covered California and the president deserve to celebrate."[44] Overall, California is a striking example of consent and perceived success that contrasts with the much more contentious situation prevailing in other states discussed later in this chapter.

Hard Cases: ACA Opponents and the Politics of Consent

It is important to note that even states that ended up rejecting any direct involve-ment in the health insurance exchanges took part in the initial discussions over the implementation of health insurance exchanges. This is true because of the initial uncertainty over the fate of the ACA and, especially, the idea that shaping the implementation process could serve the interests of all states, including those that explicitly opposed the 2010 law. Bargaining began through informal phone calls between state and federal officials, negotiations taking place between the states and the federal Center for Consumer Information and Insurance Oversight (CCIIO), and higher-profile intergovernmental conferences. For instance, on August 30, 2010, HHS hosted a one-day conference on issues regarding implementation of the exchanges. Stakeholders "discussed several aspects of exchange implementation, from the needs of consumers and employers to general operations, including eligibility and enrollment of participants, plan qualifications, and the role of the Exchanges in promoting delivery system reform."[45] State officials participated in the conference, and several of them appeared as featured speakers in panels on meeting consumer needs, qualified plans and design, operation of exchanges, and enrollment and eligibility. In the following years, CCIIO organized conferences gathering state and federal officials to discuss implementation issues regarding health insurance exchanges.[46] States that later decided to let HHS create exchanges within their borders participated in such conferences and sometimes even discussed plans to implement their own exchanges, which never materialized. For instance, at a CCIIO meeting held in Denver in May 2011, Wisconsin, a state in which Republican governor Scott Walker ended up rejecting state-run exchanges a year and a half later, presented a detailed plan about how it would implement such exchanges.[47] This example points to the fact that, even in states that ultimately decided not to implement their own exchanges, officials discussed this possibility extensively with federal officials and other state health-policy colleagues.

Six months earlier, in December 2010, "150 officials from more than 45 states" had met "with federal officials to map plans for creation of the exchanges."[48] What emerged was a pattern of reluctant consent and cooperation in a context of high policy and political uncertainty. As the *New York Times* reported, "Many state officials, including governors and state legislators, are reluctantly making plans to comply with the federal law even as they denounce it. They gave two reasons for these seemingly contradictory actions. States can obtain hundreds of millions of dollars in federal grants under the law, and they want to overhaul their own insurance markets."[49] Regarding the first issue, federal implementation grants, nearly all states received the early basic planning grant, and more than thirty-five states received a Level 1 establishment grant, a clear sign of early consent or, at least, of a willingness to explore cooperation on the part of a majority of the states, including Republican-controlled ones.[50] As Figure 3.1 shows, there is a strong correlation between the partisan composition of state legislatures and the level of exchange grant funds returned to HHS. States with unified Democratic governments returned vir-

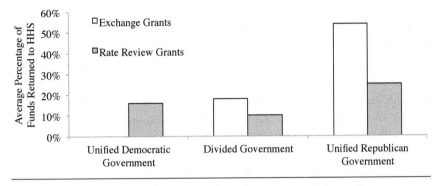

Figure 3.1 State Partisan Composition and Grant Funds Returned to HHS

Note: N = 47. Excludes Alaska (took no funds), Nebraska (Republican governor and nonpartisan legislature), and Rhode Island (independent governor and Democratic legislature). The denominator is all grants received. State partisan control refers to the date when grant funds were returned. Partisan control in Iowa, Kansas, Louisiana, Mississippi, New Jersey, New Mexico, South Carolina, and Virginia reflects 2011 off-cycle or special-election results.

Source: Compiled by authors from Government Accountability Office, *Patient Protection and Affordable Care Act: HHS's Process for Awarding and Overseeing Exchange and Rate Review Grants to States,* GAO-15-543, May 2013. Partisan control data compiled by authors from Ballotpedia.com.

tually none of their exchange planning and establishment grants, whereas states where Republicans controlled at least one legislative chamber or the governorship returned on average 18 percent of their grant funds. States with unified Republican control returned, on average, 54 percent of these funds. By way of comparison, Figure 3.1 shows that the same partisan pattern cannot be found in states' return of grants for improving the review of premium rate increases. Chapter 5 will discuss the reasons for this difference in greater detail.

Another piece of evidence regarding the logic of consent at work in many states after the enactment of the ACA is the adoption by the National Association of Insurance Commissioners (NAIC) of a model law for state exchanges. Known as the American Health Benefit Exchange Model Act, this model law "provides a basic statutory framework designed to comply with" the ACA's mandates.[51] The NAIC's move reflected the fact that, at the time, even states participating in court challenges to the ACA said they were "moving forward to plan for the insurance exchanges."[52] These remarks point to the central role of consent and cooperation in the early stages of the implementation process.

Through the NAIC, all states participated in discussions with the HHS regarding the implementation of health insurance exchanges. For instance, in a letter sent to the Centers for Medicare and Medicaid Services (CMS) in October 2011, the NAIC offered detailed comments on the HHS's Proposed Rule on the Establishment of Exchanges and Qualified Health Plans. Before offering detailed feedback on these rules, the NAIC's letter, signed by the insurance commissioners of Iowa, Florida, Louisiana, and North Dakota, stated, "In the spirit of state-federal cooperation, we have several suggestions . . . to help ensure that Exchanges deliver on the statute's promise of a transformed marketplace that streamlines the purchase of health insurance and allows consumers to make better informed decisions regarding their coverage."[53] Such an explicit emphasis on cooperation points to the logic of negotiated consent mentioned above.

Considerable discussion between state and HHS officials took place over proposed federal rules regarding the implementation of the exchanges. Evidence of this type of interaction is ever present in the comments by state officials and other stakeholders during the formulation of HHS's Proposed Rule on the Establishment of Exchanges and Qualified Health Plans. With their comments, state officials, even those from jurisdictions formally opposed to the ACA, attempted to shape the content of the proposed rule of implementation. For example, in late October 2011, the commissioner of insurance of Kansas, a state that ultimately rejected the idea of state-run exchanges after establishing several exchange working groups,[54] wrote to HHS to provide detailed and constructive feedback about the proposed rule before emphasizing the autonomy of the state in deciding how to proceed concerning the establishment of exchanges within its borders: "Kansas stakeholders have spent thousands of hours studying the options available to Kansas, and their recommendations should form the policy foundation of any Kansas exchange."[55] Tennessee, another red state, seriously studied the possibility of adopting state-run exchanges before letting the federal government act alone.[56] The state also provided detailed feedback on the proposed rule through a letter sent by its Department of Finance and Administration, Division of Health Care Finance and Administration.[57] Interestingly, the letter shows how different states collaborated to provide feedback to HHS on the implementation of exchanges. As stated in that letter, Tennessee officials "worked with representatives from Arizona, Utah, and a number of other states to develop constructive recommendations for CCIIO on a number of issues that are addressed in this and other sets of proposed rules." Joint recommendations from Arizona, Tennessee, and Utah are included in an appendix to the letter. This type of cooperation among states to pressure HHS to revise its proposed rule is a significant aspect of the politics of consent and bargaining that emerged in the aftermath of the ACA's adoption.

THE POLITICS OF DISSENT

Despite the patterns of consent and federal flexibility to promote state cooperation described above, factors such as institutional fragmentation, state autonomy embedded in policy design, and mixed public sentiments about the ACA generated much state-level opposition to health care reform over time. This situation pushed a large number of states to embrace dissent and to reject the opportunity to set up their own exchanges, which increased the direct role of the federal government in the implementation of this crucial legislation. According to Simon Haeder and David Weimer, "The most conservative states—those that totally refuse to cooperate on implementation—may end up with substantially more liberal exchanges because of the leadership of the HHS."[58] Although only time will tell about the policy substance of federal versus state exchanges, the political rewards of defaulting to a federal exchange as a means of protest were more immediate.

Opponents of the ACA had the best luck fomenting dissent on exchanges in states governed by Republicans.[59] As Figure 3.2 shows, the results of statewide elections immediately following the enactment of the ACA were strong predictors of state investment in the exchanges, with Republican-controlled states generally defaulting to a federal exchange either as a way of responding to constituents hostile to reform, banking on the reform's eventual repeal, or waiting to see what other similar states were doing. Yet, as we illustrate next, and as the following chapters confirm, partisanship is not a sufficient explanation as to why the exchanges became a target for the opposition.

How Policy Legacies and Institutional Fragmentation Mattered

State decisions about health insurance exchanges were highly vulnerable to the politics of dissent. First, exchanges represented a new policy instrument in the vast majority of states. These states, however, had no prior experience in setting up such policy instruments. As a result, there were no existing legal rules, vested interests, or economic relationships that otherwise could have facilitated federal-state cooperation over the implementation of exchanges. Despite the infusion of federal resources and the willingness of HHS to be flexible to state needs, most states would have had to create *new* statutory authority—through the legislative process—in order to construct exchanges. By the time the ACA was implemented, however, exchanges were subject to "guilt by association" and Republican opposition, making legislative enactment challenging. The policy legacy associated with health insurance exchanges thus strongly contrasted with the legacies of Medicaid, a program that since 1965 has been central to intergovernmental relations across the country.

The institutional design of the exchanges was also fragmented in important ways. It gave little capacity to federal agencies to implement exchanges if states failed to do so. As a *Politico* reporter quipped, "A quirk in the Affordable Care Act is that while it gives HHS the authority to create a federal exchange for states that

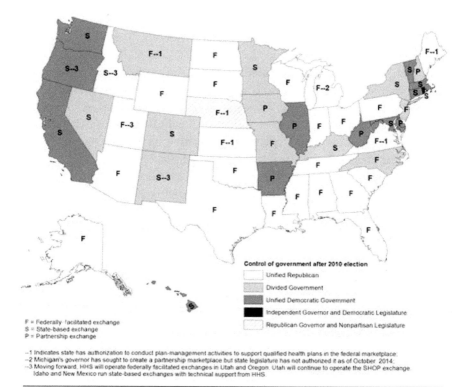

Figure 3.2 State Decisions on Health Insurance Exchanges as of April 2014

Note: Partisan control in Iowa, Kansas, Louisiana, Mississippi, New Jersey, New Mexico, South Carolina, and Virginia reflects 2011 off-cycle or special-election results.

Source: Decision data compiled by authors from Kaiser Family Foundation, "State Decisions for Creating Health Insurance Marketplaces," accessed October 25, 2014, http://kff.org/health-reform/state-indicator/state-decisions-for-creating-health-insurance-marketplaces/. Partisan control data compiled by authors from Ballotpedia.com.

don't set up their own, it doesn't actually provide any funding to do so."[60] As a consequence, because "Congress did not provide any additional discretionary funds for ACA implementation," the CMS had to rely on "funds from other sources to help pay for ongoing administrative costs associated with exchange operations."[61] Thus the federal "fallback," meant to incentivize states to create their own exchanges, did not immediately appear a credible threat. Rather, state resistance would stretch HHS's resources thin, leading to policy mishaps. As Governor Phil Bryant (R-MS) later put it, "If enough states exercise their clear and completely legal options to resist [the ACA's] implementation—including declining to establish exchanges and rejecting the Medicaid expansion—Congress will be forced to reopen the law, and a Republican-controlled House will be in a stronger position than when the law was first rammed through."[62]

Especially before the Supreme Court decision in June 2012 and the reelection of President Obama in November of that year, most GOP-controlled states had little political incentive to approve the creation of state-operated exchanges because doing so would have weakened their political and legal mobilization against the ACA.[63] The incentives the ACA provided to states—including more than $4.8 billion in grants to establish exchanges—had less capacity to secure states' consent against a tide of opposition in state capitals after the 2010 election.

Governors and state legislatures had the *opportunity* to resist because the ACA's provisions determined that exchanges were to be state "innovations." Although the law did not prevent states from creating exchanges within existing state agencies, its language suggested that exchanges were innovations states would "establish" before 2014. If exchanges were "new," they needed legislative or gubernatorial approval.[64] Entrepreneurial insurance commissioners such as Mike Chaney of Mississippi could not use their preexisting authority to create them. In fall 2013, Chaney, who was at odds with Governor Bryant on a host of issues, attempted to use his agency's preexisting authority under Mississippi law to create an exchange without gubernatorial or legislative approval. Chaney's agency worked furiously to get legal approval from the state attorney general, a Democrat.[65] The Mississippi Insurance Department created a marketing campaign for the nonexistent exchange, and Chaney himself pitched the exchange before a crowd at a Mississippi State University football game.[66] Yet this was not enough. By December, Bryant concluded that Chaney did not have the authority to construct the exchange and wrote a letter to HHS to publicly confirm his legal position on Chaney's plan.[67] Sensing a perilous fight against the governor and legislature, Chaney relented. Facing similar legal barriers, few insurance commissioners in states like Mississippi followed in his footsteps.

Broadly speaking, the ACA's opponents took advantage of the fragmented institutional structure of the exchanges, which provided few incentives for states to cooperate with the federal government. More importantly, because the vast majority of states did not already have institutions such as the exchanges, dissent simply required opponents to kill attempts at passing new legislation. Rather than creating a legislative coalition *in favor* of dissent, opponents merely needed to use the veto points in the state legislative process, which posed few collective action problems. Table 3.1 illustrates this claim by showing the process by which states established or failed to establish exchanges. Here we see that, whatever states' final decisions, most of them depended upon legislative approval. In states that did not ultimately establish exchanges, legislatures were especially reluctant to give that approval; exchange legislation introduced in these states failed to pass prior to the

Table 3.1 Pathways to State Decisions on Health Insurance Exchanges

States That Created Exchanges	
Created prior to ACA	MA, UT#
Created through gubernatorial action (executive order or declaration)	DE,* IA,* KY, NH,* NY, RI
Created through legislation	AR, CA, CO, CT, HI, ID,# IL, MD, MN, NM,# NV, OR,# VT, WA, WV*
States That Did Not Create Exchanges	
Exchange legislation introduced and failed to pass	AL, AK, AZ, FL, GA, IA, IN, KS,* ME,* NC, ND, OH,* OK, PA, SC, TX, VA,* WI
Governor announcement	LA, MS, MT,* NE,* SD,* TN, WY
Governor veto	NJ
Legislature stalled governor attempt to create partnership exchange	MI
Ballot measure to oppose exchange	MO

*Indicates state has authorization to conduct plan-management activities to support qualified health plans in the federal marketplace.

#Moving forward, HHS will operate federally facilitated exchanges in Utah and Oregon. Utah will continue to operate the SHOP exchange. Idaho and New Mexico run state-based exchanges with technical support from HHS.

governor's announcement of the state's final decision. Even in Michigan, where the governor attempted to establish partnership exchanges with the federal government, the state legislature failed to pass legislation authorizing state agencies to do so. In New Jersey, a Republican governor, Chris Christie, vetoed a bill establishing an exchange passed by a Democratic legislature. Finally, in states such as Louisiana and Wyoming, no legislators introduced bills to create exchanges.

To be sure, dissent took other forms as well. Ideologically charged and typically backed by the GOP, for instance, anti-ACA laws and resolutions enacted in many states were meant in large part to register and publicize formal political dissent against the federal reform. According to the National Conference of State Legislatures (NCSL), "between 2010 and July of 2013, 21 state legislatures had enacted laws and measures related to opting out, opposing, or seeking to challenge broad provisions of health reform, especially related to mandatory provisions of the Patient Protection and Affordable Care Act (ACA)."[68] Yet whereas largely *symbolic* legislation to nullify the individual mandate passed in eighteen states, opponents in only seven states could gather majorities to pass substantive legislation to limit state agencies' authority to implement various parts of the ACA.[69] By contrast, opponents merely had to fail to act to create exchanges, making dissent a particularly straightforward strategy.

Thus, by fall 2013, the uncertainty created by the law's provisions that allowed governors to "not lift a finger" became clear.[70] As a growing number of state governments decided not to cooperate in creating the exchanges, the administration was forced to develop federally funded health insurance exchanges in those states, and this proved hugely problematic.[71] Because the ACA had assumed states would bear the full brunt of the costs of exchange development, the law provided the federal government only a small amount of cash to develop the information technology for the program.[72] Because Republicans took control of the House in the aftermath of the 2010 midterms, it became impossible to get Congress to authorize extra funding for setting up federal exchanges, and House Republicans even attempted to defund the ACA entirely.[73] Despite the failure of such attempts, HHS remained underfunded and under pressure to develop federally funded exchanges for many more states than it had originally expected—and in a short time span. This situation also underscored the impact of Republican control of the House when that chamber refused to appropriate additional implementation funds to help HHS address this challenge.[74] When federally funded exchanges came online in October 2013—amid a budget battle that included Republican proposals to repeal the ACA—HHS was ill prepared to deal with the volume of online traffic it received. Furthermore, when the Obama administration was criticized about the law's elimination of cheaper health insurance options that did not provide minimum standards of coverage, governors in Republican states used the opportunity to levy additional political challenges to the reform. In response to this criticism, the Obama administration ultimately gave state-level officials the discretion to renew these plans through 2014—a major concession to opponents of the reform.[75]

Despite good-faith bargaining attempts on the part of HHS, difficulty with federal-state collaboration stemming from explicit political dissent could also spoil implementation efforts beyond the initial decision about whether to create state-run exchanges or not.[76] Some governors actively refused to inform citizens about the law, using their powers to prevent health insurance "navigators" from having access to information that would permit them to enroll currently uninsured individuals.[77] These actions threatened to reduce the potential enrollment of healthy individuals into health insurance exchanges, necessary for realizing the cost-reduction goals of the ACA.

Day-to-day bureaucratic relationships in policy implementation between federal and state actors, also critical to implementation, came increasingly under fire.[78] As mentioned above, the design of the law requires HHS to bargain with state executive officials over a number of rules that govern these exchanges, such as standards for essential health benefits that health care plans must cover. Republican leaders in a number of states objected to these standards, greatly hindering implementation efforts as the exchanges began to go online.[79] As a survey of state policy makers suggests, Democratic governors and their bureaucratic counterparts embraced the ACA and developed close ties with Democrats at HHS, participating in informal rule-making negotiations and staying in frequent contact; at the same time, nonpartisan bureaucrats in Republican states had more tenuous relationships with federal officials.[80] Often, Republican governors exacerbated interagency tensions by giving state policy makers a limited set of bargaining parameters on which federal agencies were not able to negotiate. As one interviewee responded, "Because of the State leadership, the relationship is strained. I feel the federal HHS has been firm and reasonable with the state while the governor has been very unreasonable and unsupportive of provided [sic] resources to poor people."[81] This quote further illustrates the existence of strong patterns of dissent in conservative, GOP-controlled states.

Importantly, these patterns of dissent were not the pure product of independent actions on the part of GOP-controlled states. This is true because, from an institutional standpoint, state opponents to the ACA discussed and even coordinated their dissent strategies through a number of bodies and networks, including the American Legislative Exchange Council (ALEC). Created in 1973, ALEC gathers "conservative state lawmakers who share a common belief in limited government, free markets, federalism, and individual liberty."[82] Operating its own Health and Human Services Task Force, ALEC has helped to coordinate state-level conservative efforts against the ACA. For instance, in 2011, ALEC issued a twenty-four-page document, *State Legislators Guide to Repealing ObamaCare,* which provided concrete advice to state officials about how to derail the implementation of the ACA. Regarding exchanges, one of the recommendations of this ALEC report was for state policy makers to refuse federal grants aimed at helping them implement state-run exchanges.[83] In addition to this report, ALEC put forward the Health Care Freedom Act, a model bill that "prohibits health insurers from accepting federal subsidies under the Affordable Care Act that trigger the employer mandate."[84] Such initiatives helped ALEC coordinate the conservative mobilization against the ACA and, more specifically, against the successful implementation of health insurance exchanges in the states. Although other conservative networks such as the Tea Party and its allies also played a direct role in the coordination of anti-ACA dissent in the states, the impact of ALEC in that area proved strong.[85]

Public Sentiments and the Importance of the Individual Mandate

Public sentiments also gave conservatives a window of opportunity to challenge the exchanges. Yet the issue here was not the way people perceived the exchanges

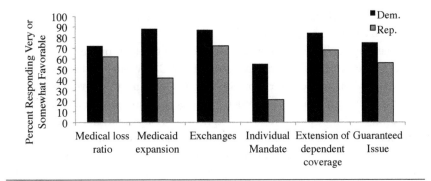

Figure 3.3 Public Support for Health Care Reform Provisions by Partisan Identification, March 2013

Source: Kaiser Family Foundation, Health Tracking Poll, March 2013, accessed June 7, 2014, http://kff.org/health-reform/poll-finding/march-2013-tracking-poll/.

in and of themselves. As suggested in Figure 3.3, support for this policy instrument was strong among both Democrats and Republicans. In this context, conservatives depicted their opposition to state-run exchanges as a symbol of their general opposition to the ACA and, more specifically, to the much less popular individual mandate, to which exchanges were perceived to be closely related. Therefore what especially mattered here was mixed public sentiments toward the ACA in general and the individual mandate in particular. Once again, the logic of "guilt by association" was at work.

Early during the implementation process, a relationship between public sentiments and the politics of implementation became clear because states where citizens held the most favorable views of the ACA in general had the greatest level of activity regarding setting up health insurance exchanges. Among the fifteen most liberal states in terms of public sentiments, for instance, only New Jersey "had not made progress beyond an initial application for an exchange establishment grant."[86] In the end, Republican governor Christie echoed mixed public sentiments in vetoing legislation by the Democrat-controlled state legislature.[87] Because of the higher support for the ACA in New Jersey, however, Governor Christie framed his second, 2012 veto as a pragmatic decision derived from the uncertainty surrounding the implementation process: "I will not ask New Jerseyans to commit today to a State-based Exchange when the federal government cannot tell us what it will cost, how that cost compares to our other options, and how much control they will give the states over this state-financed option."[88] In this particular case, partisanship and perhaps Christie's own national political ambitions trumped public sentiments, in the sense that New Jersey ended up having the federal government implement its exchange, whereas unified Democratic control would likely have resulted in a state-run exchange.

Regarding public sentiments, state decisions to run their own exchanges were central to the successful implementation of the ACA because of the impact such decisions had on public perceptions of the law's legitimacy. A governor's refusal to implement a state health insurance exchange was not only an administrative choice but a form of public dissent designed to stir up opposition to the law. In some states, governors also crafted their refusal in order to avoid blame for problems associated with the law's implementation. As Republican governor Paul Le-Page of Maine put it, "I'm not lifting a finger. . . . [Maine is] not going to get involved. We're going to let Mr. Obama do a federal exchange. It's his bill."[89] Viewed from this angle, it is clear that rejecting state-run exchanges was a way for dissident state officials to signal their opposition to the ACA and the Obama administration and attempt to weaken public support for federal health care reform.

CHOOSING A STRATEGY: THE POLITICS OF DISSENT AND CONSENT IN FOUR STATES

This broad overview of exchange implementation in the states suggests that the level of dissent varied greatly from one state to another. In order to provide a more nuanced and detailed analysis of the politics of dissent, this section briefly turns to one state that exhibited a strong level of dissent (Texas) and three states that featured a changing mix of dissent and consent that affected the degree of cooperation witnessed in these three jurisdictions (North Carolina, Arkansas, and Missouri).

Texas: Saying "No" to the Federal Government

Texas is no stranger to "saying no" to the federal government. In 2011, legislators in the Lone Star State easily passed a bill that nullified, albeit unconstitutionally, federal rules on energy-efficient lightbulbs.[90] Thus Texas provides a great political contrast with the case of California, discussed above, because the Lone Star State is much more conservative on average than the Golden State in terms of public sentiments and political culture. In Texas, lack of prior action on the establishment of insurance exchanges along with the ACA's fragmented design empowered Republicans governing the state to very publicly express their opposition to federal health care reform and to the Democratic president who signed it.

From the beginning, Texas governor Rick Perry was a strong opponent of the ACA despite the fact that his state took concrete, low-profile steps to adapt to the federal reform, as other conservative states did.[91] Largely driven by partisanship, the governor's position appeared in tension with the reality that "with the highest percentage of uninsured residents, Texas would be one of the biggest beneficiaries of President Barack Obama's health care overhaul."[92] Yet, as a prominent conservative Republican governor and a 2012 GOP presidential hopeful, Perry embraced dissent in a powerful and theatrical way, losing no opportunity to slam "Obamacare." Joining the lawsuit against the ACA, Governor Perry made it clear his state would reject both Medicaid expansion and the creation of its own health insurance exchange. In a July 2012 statement, he made his position extra clear:

> If anyone was in doubt, we in Texas have no intention to implement so-called state exchanges or to expand Medicaid under Obamacare. . . . I will not be party to socializing healthcare and bankrupting my state in direct contradiction to our Constitution and our founding principles of limited government. I stand proudly with the growing chorus of governors who reject the Obamacare power grab. Neither a "state" exchange nor the expansion of Medicaid under this program would result in better "patient protection" or in more "affordable care." They would only make Texas a mere appendage of the federal government when it comes to health care.[93]

Rooted explicitly in his defense of state autonomy and lack of trust in the federal government and the Obama administration, Perry's clear decision to let the federal government implement the health insurance exchange in Texas seemed rather paradoxical because it allowed the federal government to directly shape such an exchange instead of giving state officials the opportunity to play a much more direct role in that policy area. Here, the logic of "guilt by association" discussed above seemed at work in the sense that the health insurance exchanges became politically contaminated by their association with the ACA and the Democratic president who signed it. Governor Perry's decision to reject the ACA as a whole seemed in tune with public sentiments in his state because more people opposed the law than supported it. This presents a strong contrast with the situation prevailing in California, where the reform found more friends than skeptics.[94] Dominated by Republicans, the legislative branch in Texas adopted a similar position against the ACA and, as a consequence, health insurance exchanges. Texas-based Democrats and liberal groups criticized Governor Perry's attitude and pushed the state to create its own exchange instead of letting the federal government do so as a default option. In a state entirely controlled by Republicans, however, this push went nowhere. For instance, in early 2013, Texas Democratic representative Eric Johnson put forward a bill aimed at implementing a state-run exchange in the state, but this initiative, just like his bill supporting Medicaid expansion in Texas, went nowhere.[95] Overall, it quickly became clear that, in the name of the institutional autonomy granted by the policy design of exchanges in the context of the ACA, state officials would let the federal government take on the burden of implementing a health insurance exchange in Texas.

As in other states that decided to let Washington implement the exchanges within their borders, the federal government recruited powerful allies to help it successfully launch such an exchange in Texas. Among these allies was Blue Cross Blue Shield; in April 2013, some of its top executives had extended talks with White House officials about the federal implementation of state exchanges. In Texas as in other states, Blue Cross Blue Shield sought to protect its market shares through this alliance with the Obama administration, which needed as much support as possible to advertise for and promote enrollment in the health insurance exchanges it created in states dominated by antagonistic Republican officials. Pushing to get uninsured individuals from Texas to enroll, Blue Cross Blue Shield launched a systematic campaign to reach out to them. As Michelle Riddell, vice president of community investment for Blue Cross Blue Shield of Texas, told a reporter: "In campaign terms, it's a get-out-the-vote type of approach."[96] Because the public in Texas, as elsewhere in the country, had limited knowledge of how the exchanges would work, and the state government strongly opposed the ACA, Blue Cross Blue Shield of Texas played a direct role in "educating and recruiting exchange customers with little cooperation from the state."[97] This is an example of how the Obama administration managed to get allies on board to facilitate its task in implementing the exchanges in states such as Texas characterized by high levels of political dissent.

However, dissent is seldom absolute, and there is evidence that even in Texas, state policies may have helped the federal government stimulate enrollment in the health insurance exchanges Governor Perry and his conservative allies had so strongly condemned in the name of their systematic opposition to the ACA and the Obama administration's agenda. For instance, in 2013, Texas decided to "shut down its high-risk insurance pool for some of the state's sickest residents, pushing participants to find private coverage in the federal health insurance marketplace created under the federal Affordable Care Act."[98] Although this change only concerned 23,000 people, it suggests that, after the June 2012 Supreme Court decision to uphold most of the ACA, along with the November reelection of President Obama, officials in Texas took for granted the fact that this "law of the land" would apply to their state despite the heated rhetoric from their governor about the need to repeal it. As the chapter on regulation suggests, this basic form of pragmatism was present in other high-dissent states explicitly opposed to the ACA but forced to live with it somehow. Yet, as far as the health insurance exchanges are concerned, the *explicit* level of collaboration in the field of regulation is seldom visible in Texas, perhaps in part because exchanges have a much higher political profile—and public visibility—than regulatory policy.

Despite Governor Perry's vocal opposition to the ACA, by March 2014 nearly 750,000 people in Texas "had obtained private insurance through the Marketplace. Of these, 225,000 (30.2%) were previously uninsured. Although a seemingly small proportion of Texans obtained insurance through the state's Marketplace, the large absolute numbers had a substantial impact on increasing access to insurance coverage in the United States."[99] In other words, despite the initial problems with the HealthCare.gov website, in Texas just as elsewhere in the United States, the new exchange started to make a difference, notwithstanding the high level of dissent prevailing in the Lone Star State and in other conservative, GOP-controlled states.

North Carolina: When a Partisan Switch Means Stalled Reform

North Carolina, a large red state with nearly 10 million inhabitants, further illustrates the impact of partisanship on the politics of implementation. This politics was made possible by the institutional context of federalism and the policy design of the ACA, which gave power to the states to decide whether to create their own exchanges—power that became more real because of mixed public sentiments about the federal health insurance reform. From this perspective, the story of North Carolina is about not only partisanship but also the institutional and public opinion conditions under which a swift shift from consent to dissent was possible and meaningful in the first place.

When the ACA became law in March 2010, the governor of North Carolina was Democrat Bev Purdue. Purdue was elected in November 2008, at the same time Obama won the presidential race. This meant, in the months following the adoption of the ACA, North Carolina seemed on track to implement a state-run health insurance exchange because preparations were under way for the state to move forward instead of letting the federal government fulfill this task. Yet, the governor's task was severely complicated when, in the aftermath of the 2010 state elections, Republicans gained majority control of the state legislature's lower and upper chambers. In this context, a "bill authorizing an exchange cleared the House" but "did not pass in the Senate."[100] In the 2012 gubernatorial elections, after a campaign in which ACA implementation appeared a significant topic, Republican Pat McCrory won easily with about 55 percent of the vote. McCrory defeated Democrat Walter Dalton, who had won his party's nomination after Governor Purdue announced she would not seek a second term. In 2012, Republicans also won majorities in both legislative chambers, which gave the "GOP unified control of the North Carolina government for the first time since 1870."[101] In the aftermath of these electoral outcomes, it became clear that the partnership exchange Governor Purdue had openly contemplated before the 2012 elections would not materialize. In fact, the following year, a new law rejected both the expansion of Medicaid and the creation of a health insurance exchange by the state and returned "more than $20 million in federal funds previously awarded to North Carolina to help establish an exchange."[102] This decision to return previously awarded federal funds to facilitate the implementation of health insurance exchanges by the state was not unique to North Carolina because other backtracking states did exactly the same thing.[103] Interestingly, North Carolina insurance commissioner Wayne Goodwin criticized that decision and the new legislation: "Having a federal exchange in North Carolina will no doubt limit our ability to resolve consumers' health insurance issues at the state level. . . . People who have questions, concerns, or complaints about health insurance will have to seek out help from the federal government rather than from trusted regulators in our own state."[104] Governor McCrory stated he would have preferred the state to implement its own health insurance exchange, but there was too much uncertainty surrounding the ACA to ensure that the state would enjoy adequate autonomy to shape the exchange according to the state's own needs. He concluded that this was "not an easy decision," a statement that contrasts with the powerful rhetoric of Governor Perry quoted above.[105] The North Carolina GOP governor's more nuanced discourse might simply be related to the fact that his state was not nearly as conservative as some other southern states. For instance, in the 2012 presidential election, Romney barely won the state with a two-point lead over Obama, a situation that contrasted with the one in Texas, in which Romney won with a more than fifteen-point lead over his Democratic opponent.

Regardless, after the 2012 state elections, because "both legislative and executive branches of North Carolina government publicly eschewed involvement in the ACA, . . . the state insurance department could do nothing to help its marketplace achieve success. Grassroots efforts and the generic federally run website were the entire public face of the HIM [Health Insurance Marketplace] in North Carolina."[106] Among these grassroots efforts, the nonprofit organization Enroll America played a direct role in North Carolina. By purchasing advertisements to stimulate enrollment in the federally organized North Carolina exchanges, Enroll America complemented the efforts of the federal government. Simultaneously, as in Texas and other red states that refused to implement their own exchanges largely in order to distance themselves from the ACA, there was "no state-organized outreach and enrollment effort, no state campaign to raise awareness about new coverage options, and no state-led drive to cover hard-to-reach populations such as immigrants."[107] Overall, after contemplating the possibility and even trying to pass legislation aimed at implementing a state-run health insurance exchange under Governor Purdue, North Carolina made a policy U-turn, triggered in large part by changes in the electoral landscape as a result of Republican gains in both 2010 and 2012, when McCrory won the gubernatorial race for the GOP.

Despite the lack of state support in terms of implementation, in North Carolina, according to an Urban Institute study released in May 2014, more than 350,000 people signed up for exchange-based coverage, and, as a consequence, "North Carolina hit 145 percent of its goal, the second highest percentage of any of the 34 states that accessed the federally facilitated marketplace, healthcare.gov."[108] In other words, the federally run exchange proved popular in North Carolina despite the strong GOP opposition that gradually pushed the state to openly reject the ACA and the implementation of a state-run exchange. Another sign of departure from the unilateral, Tea Party–like political stance of the North Carolina GOP about the ACA is that, according to an April 2014 New York Times Upshot/Kaiser Family Foundation poll, 60 percent of respondents from that state preferred to see the law improved rather than terminated.[109] That poll also revealed significantly stronger support for this idea in North Carolina than in Kentucky and Louisiana, two other southern states in which public sentiments toward the ACA were more negative on average.[110] This is partly why North Carolina is a hybrid case in contrast with more conservative states such as Texas.

Arkansas: Divided Government and the Politics of Partnership

Arkansas reacted differently to the ACA than many other conservative, southern states, a situation related to the presence in 2010 of both a Democratic governor and a "strongly Democratic legislature."[111] Although Democrats lost many seats in the 2010 state elections, they remained in control of both the Arkansas House and Senate. Moreover, Democratic governor Mike Beebe was easily reelected for a second mandate in November 2010 with approximately 65 percent of the votes. In the aftermath of the 2012 state elections, however, Republicans took control of the state's House and Senate, a key development that further complicated the political situation of Governor Beebe, who generally supported the idea of cooperating with the federal government regarding the ACA, an approach that strongly contrasted with the typical Republican opposition to cooperation and the implementation of a state-led exchange in Arkansas. These developments point to the role of institutional fragmentation at the state level, which allowed conservative opposition to the ACA to mobilize against the potential advent of state-run exchanges in a context of mixed public sentiments and a policy design that allowed states to pass on the opportunity to bring about such exchanges without direct financial loss, in contrast to the situation prevailing in the field of Medicaid expansion.

As in other states, observers pointed to the paradoxical nature of the GOP opposition to a state-run health insurance exchange in Arkansas: "It may seem

strange that conservatives, usually strongly in favor of more state control, have led
the charge against state-run exchanges, seemingly ceding more authority to the
federal government.... [This] opposition to state-run exchanges is part of the platform of continued resistance to the ACA that animates the Republican base."[112]
From this perspective, in Arkansas as in many other states, GOP opposition to
state-run exchanges was part of a broader dissent strategy meant to weaken the
implementation of the ACA across the country and publicly display open resistance to it. It was also a way to appeal to the conservative and Tea Party base. Once
again, mixed public sentiments as well as the policy design of the ACA and the
institutional logic of state autonomy within a fragmented federal system made this
strategy possible in the first place.

In this broad institutional and political context, in 2011, even before the GOP
took control of the Arkansas House and the Senate, systematic opposition from
Republicans helped prevent the adoption of legislation allowing the creation of a
state-run exchange. As one commentator noted, "Unified Republican opposition
to state control beat the more sensible idea of taking federal planning money so
that Arkansas insurance regulators could set up a plan tailored to Arkansas. Yes,
Republicans are in the minority in the legislature, barely. But they were prepared
to hammer every Democrat on the ballot with Obamacare had the money been
taken."[113] Thus, in this conservative state, well-organized Republicans played a
crucial role even before they seized control of the state legislature after the 2012
elections.

In fall 2012, Governor Beebe officially opted for the recently created, post-ACA
partnership exchange model, according to which the state would help the federal
government implement and run health insurance exchanges in Arkansas.[114] In a
letter to HHS secretary Kathleen Sebelius, Governor Beebe requested approval to
take over from the federal government both consumer assistance and plan management, claiming that the creation of such a partnership exchange would "place
Arkansas in a good position to make the transition to a State-Based Exchange in the
future should legislative authority be obtained to do so."[115] This statement clearly
implied the quest for greater state autonomy in the future because the partnership
approach was described as a potential road to the advent of state-run exchanges.
The following month, in an interview with the Associated Press, Governor Beebe
confirmed his hope to move forward with an entirely state-run exchange system in
the future: "Right now the Legislature has indicated no desire to change anything
to go to a pure state-run (exchange). So we'll continue where we are and they'll
continue to gather information, and when and if I get a consensus or expression
from the Legislature that they want . . . a state exchange, then we'll write another
letter."[116] To justify the idea of a partnership exchange, Governor Beebe deployed
the traditional rhetoric about state autonomy frequently associated with the GOP:

"The State of Arkansas wishes to retain as much control and autonomy as possible with regard to the operation of our health insurance exchange, rather than concede that control to Washington, D.C."[117] In the end, along with Illinois, Iowa, Michigan, New Hampshire, and West Virginia, Arkansas became one of the first six states to enter a partnership exchange.[118]

In early 2013, however, Republican opposition to a state-run exchange declined rapidly after Governor Beebe succeeded in getting HHS to approve his private option for Medicaid, discussed in the next chapter.[119] In the context of this clear political victory for the Democratic governor, the GOP-dominated legislative branch adopted a law authorizing the "transition of the Marketplace from a state-federal Partnership Marketplace to a State-based Marketplace to take effect on July 1, 2015."[120] Governor Beebe signed the law in April 2013. From September 2013 to April 2014, during the nationwide enrollment period, 43,446 people in Arkansas selected a plan available through the Arkansas Health Insurance Marketplace, which represented about 19 percent of the potentially eligible population.[121] Such results were achieved in the context of a partnership model because the state-run system only came to life in 2015.

Missouri: Obamacare at the Ballot Box

Traditionally described as a swing state, Missouri is increasingly seen as a red state given that Obama lost by only a slight margin (against John McCain) in 2008, but by a much larger margin (against Romney) in 2012.[122] In this context, support for the ACA proved mixed at best, although some elements of the reform, such as the expansion of Medicaid, received significant popular support.[123] As will be seen below, in addition to basic factors such as state autonomy and the policy design of the ACA, allowing states to reject implementation of their own exchanges, the existence of referendum initiatives appears to have been a clear and powerful institutional factor. It empowered opponents of state-run exchanges in a context of mixed public sentiments about the health care reform and declining support for President Obama, as seen in the different results in the 2008 and 2012 presidential elections.

Despite Obama's defeats, however, Missouri did elect a Democratic governor, Jay Nixon, in 2008 by a nineteen-point margin. Nixon secured reelection in 2012, although on that occasion he only beat his Republican opponent by a twelve-point margin. At the same time, however, Republicans have controlled the Missouri Senate and House of Representatives without interruption since 2001 and 2003, respectively. During the period under analysis, the GOP remained dominant in both legislative bodies, which considerably reduced Governor Nixon's leverage in terms of the implementation of a health insurance exchange in his state. In fact, in summer 2010, the GOP put forward Proposition C (the Health Care Freedom Act), a referendum initiative that received strong support at the ballot box, where more than 70 percent of voters backed it. A symbolic and political gesture opposed by Democrats, including Governor Nixon, the Health Care Freedom Act formally authorized the state to opt out of the ACA.[124]

Despite this setback, using his institutional autonomy, the Democratic governor took steps to pave the way for the advent of a state-run health insurance exchange in Missouri, notably through the establishment of a state health insurance exchange coordinating council that "included executive leadership from multiple state agencies and established four work groups to address exchange components, including Operations, Finance and Coverage, Communications, and Cost-containment and Quality. The Council identified a number of consultants to provide background research and insurance market analysis to inform decision-making in the state."[125] In June 2011, the state Senate also created the Senate Interim Committee on health insurance exchanges to "explore Missouri's options to establish a state-based exchange."[126] Simultaneously, opposition to state-run exchanges manifested itself within the legislative branch, especially in the Senate, which led to the defeat in 2011 and 2012 of legislative initiatives meant to create such an exchange in Missouri. Interestingly, one of these initiatives came from GOP representative Chris Molendorp; his initiative "passed with no opposition in the state House but hit a wall in the Senate."[127] This means that, early on, a number of Republican officials actively supported a state-run exchange in Missouri, a position consistent with that of Governor Nixon.

In late May 2012, a few weeks before the Supreme Court decision on the ACA, to prevent Governor Nixon and the rest of the state executive branch from acting unilaterally concerning an exchange, the GOP-controlled Missouri General Assembly included a referendum on the 2012 ballot through the adoption of Senate Bill 464. The following question was asked of voters: "Shall Missouri Law be amended to prohibit the Governor, or any state agency, from establishing or operating state-based health insurance exchanges unless authorized by a vote of the people or by the legislature?" Instead of preventing the creation of a state-run exchange altogether, if passed, Proposition E would forbid the executive branch from acting unilaterally on that matter, among other things.[128] As the Missouri Foundation for Health noted,

> Proposition E prohibits establishing, creating, or operating a health insurance exchange in Missouri without a legislative act, an initiative petition, or [a] referendum authorizing the establishment and operation of the exchange. The measure expressly bars Missouri's Governor from establishing an exchange through an executive order. Proposition E outlaws all state agency activities

to implement an exchange unless authorized by statute and prohibits agencies from establishing exchange programs or issuing exchange rules or policies. State agencies are barred from performing exchange functions without statutory authority.[129]

Importantly, Proposition E also restricted the development of "federally run exchanges in Missouri by preventing state agencies from entering into agreements to establish or operate a federally facilitated exchange and from providing assistance or resources related to the creation of a federal exchange, unless the agency receives statutory authority or the assistance is mandated by federal law."[130] From this perspective, Proposition E complicated the task of the federal government in implementing an exchange in Missouri by limiting the level of cooperation between federal and state officials in that crucial policy area. Backed by Republicans and the Tea Party, this referendum initiative created a strong political challenge for Governor Nixon, who ended up adopting a neutral stance in the debate over it. Long before the November 2012 ballot, the Democratic governor had clearly stated that "his administration would not move to set up an insurance exchange by decree."[131] Yet, at the same time, other ACA supporters criticized the November 2012 referendum initiative as pure and simple political posturing on the part of opponents of the federal legislation. For instance, one prominent Missouri advocate of the ACA declared, "Prop E is really just an attempt to continue to use health care reform for political gain because there's really going to be no practical effect because health reform, the Affordable Care Act, is the law of the land."[132] Representative Molendorp, who had sponsored a 2011 bill requesting the creation of a state-run exchange in Missouri, declared that a victory of the "Yes" camp at the November referendum would simply mean that the legislature should take the initiative and bring about such an exchange by adopting a law designed for that purpose. "We have, I think, a very legitimate reason to set up our own unique exchange tailored to the complexities of the Missouri health care [system] and the Missouri insurance market."[133] This reinforced the idea that the referendum was simply about preventing the Democratic governor from acting unilaterally rather than discarding the possibility of a state-run exchange altogether. In the end, on November 6, Proposition E received nearly 62 percent of the vote, thereby killing any possibility for Governor Nixon to implement a state-run exchange by executive order and illustrating enduringly mixed public sentiments about the ACA.[134]

Less than two weeks later, the Democratic governor sent a letter to Sebelius telling her his state would not implement its own exchange.[135] In his letter, Governor Nixon clearly expressed his support for a state-run exchange in Missouri:

> We believe that regulation of the insurance market is a power best left in
> the hands of states. Since 1869, the Missouri Department of Insurance has

fostered a fair, competitive, and healthy insurance market in Missouri and protected our consumers. Further, in 2011, our General Assembly took initial steps toward establishing a state-based exchange through legislation that was passed unanimously by the House of Representatives and a Senate committee. Unfortunately, the General Assembly ultimately failed to pass that legislation. We continue to favor state, rather than federal, control of our insurance market.[136]

In contrast with Governor Nixon's wish, in 2013 and 2014 the federal government implemented the health insurance exchange in Missouri. In early August 2013, only a few months before enrollment began, the *New York Times* commented on the extremely low profile of the implementation process in Missouri: "Looking for the new health insurance marketplace, set to open in this state in two months, is like searching for a unicorn. The marketplace, or exchange, being established by the federal government under President Obama's health care law has no visible presence here, no local office, no official voice in the state, and no board of local advisers. It is being run like a covert operation, with no marketing or detailed information about its products or their prices."[137] In a state with more than 850,000 uninsured in 2013, the advent of such an exchange represented a major policy task left entirely to the federal government. Advocates of the exchange had to struggle in a changing policy environment in which improvisation became the rule in the total absence of information communicated by the state of Missouri, which remained silent over the implementation of the federally run exchange there. The president of the Missouri Hospital Association commented, "It's like running an obstacle course every day of the week, but the course changes from day to day."[138] To further complicate implementation of the ACA in in the state, in early 2014 the Missouri Senate began discussing SB 546, which would "update the Health Care Freedom Act passed by Missouri voters in 2010" to "effectively cripple the implementation of the Affordable Care Act within the state."[139] On a much more positive note for supporters of the ACA, in January 2014 a federal judge temporarily blocked a state law that imposed restrictions on the navigators tasked with helping people use the health insurance marketplace.[140] By March 11, 2014, more than 74,000 Missourians had purchased health insurance coverage through the federally run exchange.[141]

CONCLUSION

A market-friendly idea supported by prominent Republicans when it was rather uncontroversial before the adoption of the ACA, health insurance exchanges became victim to "guilt by association." Conservative opponents of the Obama administration and health insurance reform in the states attacked this previously consensual policy instrument to publicly express their dissent and directly undermine the implementation of the 2010 federal legislation. The logic of "guilt by association," along with conservative, GOP mobilization against state-run exchanges, was related to policy visibility and the high public profile of exchanges as policy instruments, especially when compared with the regulatory instruments discussed in the next chapter. Like Medicaid expansion, state-run exchanges became a highly visible and contentious target of political mobilization on the part of those seeking to reverse or at least weaken health care reform in the states during the Obama years, both before and after his 2012 reelection.

At the same time, because of their policy legacy and institutional fragmentation, state-run exchanges necessitated new positive action by state governments— enabling opponents to dissent by "not lifting a finger." Additionally, the ACA provided little in the way of either fiscal inducements or regulatory punishments for not creating exchanges, which means no tempting fiscal "carrot" or "stick" is available to sway state officials who may dislike the ACA but face direct pressure to accept a "good deal" offered by the federal government. With weak financial incentives beyond implementation subsidies, exchanges are even more prone to dissent than Medicaid expansion, which is much more attractive to the states from a strictly financial standpoint. Finally, from an institutional perspective, the decision of the US Senate to give the states the option to run their own exchanges or let the federal government create them allowed for such a high level of dissent to emerge, especially in more conservative, GOP-controlled states. In the end, health insurance exchanges became the most dissent-prone of the three policy areas under investigation because of the interaction between weak policy legacies, institutional fragmentation, and the high-profile nature of the exchanges combined with mixed public sentiments about the individual mandate and the ACA as a whole. Here, the high level of political dissent against the ACA at the state level certainly contributed to eroding the apparent legitimacy of the law and, consequently, public support for health care reform and the Obama administration, so directly associated with it.

4. Medicaid Expansion: Take It or Leave It

Medicaid is the largest and most complex federal-state program in existence.[1] In fact, by the time the Patient Protection and Affordable Care Act (ACA) was debated in Congress, Medicaid had "developed into the largest medical insurance plan in the United States."[2] Along with the associated Children's Health Insurance Program (CHIP), Medicaid provided health insurance coverage to more than 60 million Americans.[3]

As enacted, the ACA significantly increased the federal government's role in funding and organizing Medicaid, with all states expected to expand their programs to cover everyone with incomes up to 133 percent (and effectively 138 percent) of the federal poverty line (FPL) and to maintain their already existing Medicaid efforts. The scale and nature of the expansion suggested that any major reform to Medicaid would need intricate negotiation among many different political actors. Yet not long after the ACA's enactment, mobilized opposition at the state level threatened to undermine negotiations. The American Legislative Exchange Council (ALEC) *State Legislators Guide to Repealing ObamaCare* (2011) advised state legislators to dissent from the Medicaid expansion because it would "mire states" in a poorly designed program that would lead to "untenable state budgets."[4]

Though the Medicaid expansion has a longer legacy of federal-state cooperation than the health insurance exchanges and was initially less institutionally fragmented, it remains a subject of partisan and ideological contestation. This constellation of factors has produced a mix of dissent, in the form of a Supreme Court challenge and state refusals to expand the program, and consent, in the form of alternative versions of the expansion adopted by states with Republican or divided government.

At first blush, state adoption of the Medicaid expansion did not seem like an especially controversial issue, given that it demanded only small increases in states' fiscal obligations. As envisioned by the ACA's framers, the federal government would fund all the costs of expansion for the first three years, starting in 2014, with its contribution tapering down to 90 percent for all newly eligible enrollees from 2019 onward. That honeypot incentive was designed to attract state governments, but it was backed up by potentially prohibitive sanctions against any state that opted to turn its back on this federal largesse. Technically, as with the Medicaid program itself, states could refuse to participate in the expansion, but the ACA stated that in doing so they would forfeit all existing federal Medicaid funding. Hence, if the Medicaid expansion had taken place exactly as planned in the legislation signed in March 2010, although states would likely have varied in how enthusiastically they worked to enroll the newly eligible individuals and develop the administrative capacity to manage the extra caseload, they would have had little choice but to act in accordance with the ACA. In contrast to the implementation of health insurance exchanges, which always left room for states to dissent from the expectations of the ACA's framers, as written in 2010, the ACA did not provide realistic leeway for governors and state legislators to rebut the Medicaid expansion.

President Barack Obama himself explained why he thought it best that the federal government, rather than the states, take the lead in the Medicaid expansion. In an interview with David Remnick for the *New Yorker* magazine, Obama acknowledged that some conservatives genuinely saw the federal government as overly bureaucratic and unaccountable but added that the call for "states' rights" had not always served an honorable cause. So although progressives should treat conservative concerns about federal overreach as legitimate,

> the flip side is I think it's important for conservatives to recognize and answer some of the problems that are posed by that history, so that they understand if I am concerned about leaving it up to states to expand Medicaid that it may not simply be because I am this power-hungry guy in Washington who wants to crush states' rights but, rather, because we are one country and I think it is going to be important for the entire country to make sure that poor folks in Mississippi and not just Massachusetts are healthy.[5]

Opponents of health care reform did not agree, nor did the Supreme Court in its *National Federation of Independent Business (NFIB) v. Sebelius* decision in 2012. The fact that when the expansion came into effect in January 2014 there were twenty-four states, including Mississippi, that did not participate in the expansion was a direct consequence of the Supreme Court's opinion in the case that the federal government could not impose the sanction of withdrawing existing federal Medicaid funding.[6]

This verdict meant that the justices had effectively amended the institutional design of the ACA, empowering state-level opponents of the law.[7] Those states that opted out of the expansion did potentially forfeit billions of dollars, but as we will see through this chapter, the Court's ruling gave states the chance to "dissent" from the intent of the ACA, as in the case of the health insurance exchanges.[8] In fact, the dissent with regard to Medicaid had more profound effects for a state's citizens than was the case when it dissented from setting up its own insurance marketplace. When a state refused to build its own exchange, the ACA did have a "Plan B": the federal government would, however uncertainly, step in to organize an exchange on behalf of that state. This means that determined, eligible citizens in all states have an exchange to turn to and subsidies to access. When states have refused to expand their Medicaid programs, however, there has been no further federal intervention to help residents who would have gained health insurance coverage had the state expanded its program. Those who crafted the ACA did not develop a Plan B with regard to dissent from the Medicaid clauses in the bill because they never seriously considered that there would be any dissent from Plan A.

Although the Supreme Court decision, by removing the sanctions contained in the ACA, gave states the opportunity to opt out of the Medicaid expansion, the Court did not disqualify the incentives contained in the law. Therefore, even state governments run by Republicans ideologically hostile to President Obama and opposed to the principles behind the ACA faced the temptation of an influx of federal dollars. In reality, those dollars had an appeal beyond governors' mansions and state legislative chambers because they were attractive to powerful vested interests, such as hospitals, that would expect to see a reduction in the cost of uncompensated care if Medicaid covered all poor people. Further complicating matters for state political leaders who wanted to opt out of the expansion was the concern they would be vulnerable to the charge that the people of their state would be paying federal taxes to fund health insurance for people in other states but not in their own.

Despite the apparently compelling reasons for taking the federal money and expanding Medicaid, most states with unified Republican government after the 2010 midterm election had not, as of September 2014, taken part in the expansion (see Figure 4.1). In contrast to states with some level of Republican control, all states with unified Democratic government had expanded their Medicaid programs, as had some with divided partisan control.

It would, however, be oversimplifying the issue to portray the politics of the Medicaid expansion only in partisan terms. Partisan patterns do explain much but not all of the behavior and the variation in outcomes across the states. Although emphasizing the importance of partisanship, Lawrence Jacobs and Timothy Callaghan suggest that state "affluence, past policy trajectories, and administrative capacity may influence state adoption of Medicaid."[9] Certainly some states diverged from a purely partisan norm. For example, four states with unified Republican government—Arizona, Michigan, North Dakota, and Ohio—had agreed to use the federal dollars to cover the target population by the start of 2014; they were joined in August 2014 by Pennsylvania. In other cases, states with Republican or divided government engaged in a potentially "high-stakes game of intergovernmental 'chicken'" by seeking waivers giving them the policy flexibility to implement the expansion in their own particular fashion.[10]

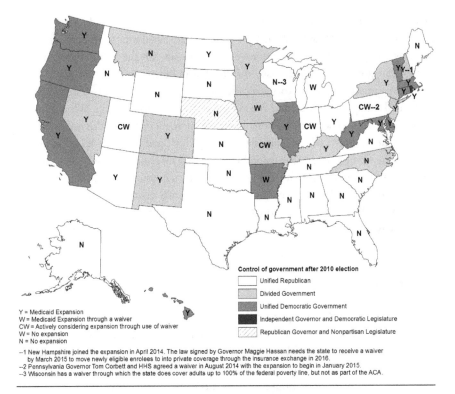

Figure 4.1 State Decisions on Medicaid Expansion as of April 2014

Note: Partisan control in Iowa, Kansas, Louisiana, Mississippi, New Jersey, New Mexico, South Carolina, and Virginia reflects 2011 off-cycle or special-election results.

Source: Decision data compiled by authors from Kaiser Family Foundation, "Status of State Action on the Medicaid Expansion Decision," accessed November 10, 2014, http://kff.org/health-reform/state-indicator/state-activity-around-expanding-medicaid-under-the-affordable-care-act/. Partisan control data compiled by authors from Ballotpedia.com.

In this chapter we show that the mixed pattern of consent and dissent in the case of Medicaid expansion can be explained by the unique configuration of policy legacies, institutional fragmentation, and public sentiments that shaped opponents' efforts to contest the reform in the states. After detailing major policy issues associated with the expansion, we illustrate how longer legacies of state innovation and gubernatorial control, coupled with juicy fiscal incentives, created a more hospitable environment for the expansion in some Republican states, whereas sharp partisan divisions on the issue incentivized opponents of the reform to engage in dissent. To illustrate the various responses to the prospect of expanding Medicaid, we track events in five states. In two of these states—California and Arizona—the expansion took place but within very different political environments. The former saw a largely enthusiastic embrace of expansion, but the latter, under unified Republican government, witnessed a bitter battle between Governor Jan Brewer and most Republican legislators. We will then examine events in two Republican-controlled states that dissented but again with some interesting differences. In Texas, Governor Rick Perry was one of the most vocal critics of the notion of expanding the program, but in Florida, Governor Rick Scott flip-flopped in his public stance as he first opposed expansion before saying he could not deny the state the money being offered before he was beaten back by a hostile state legislature, which killed the proposal. Finally, we look at Arkansas, with divided control of the state government; there, the state negotiated a deal whereby it used the money to insure those newly eligible through private insurance rather than traditional Medicaid.

POLICY ISSUES

Expanding Medicaid was a principal way in which the ACA was intended to reduce the number of uninsured in the United States. For reform advocates the Medicaid expansion helped fulfill one of their "central" goals, "to provide the quickest expansion of coverage to low-income Americans."[11] The idea of expanding Medicaid to insure more poor households as a means of getting closer to universal coverage was not new. It had been a central element of the Massachusetts reform plan in 2006.[12] Prior to this, both academic commentators on health policy and health care lobbyists had advocated Medicaid expansion as a politically practical means of reducing levels of the uninsured. For example, Lawrence Brown and Michael Sparer argued that by building on previous incremental expansions of Medicaid eligibility, policy makers could potentially edge the United States toward a "model of universal coverage" that would remain "sufficiently distinct to fit with America's stubborn exceptionalism."[13] In 2001, leading figures from Families USA and the Health Insurers Association of America (HIAA), two interest groups that had campaigned on opposite sides during the battle over the Clinton plan, came together to endorse a plan that included an expansion of Medicaid to cover everyone with an income below 133 percent of the FPL.[14]

This template, however, did not explain where the funding for the expanded coverage would come from. As discussed below, Medicaid had been placing an ever-increasing strain on state budgets, almost to a breaking point. This was especially acute in 2009 and 2010 as state finances reeled from the impact of the recession, and Medicaid rolls grew as unemployment rose. Hence the nation's governors watched anxiously through 2009 as lawmakers in Washington, DC, designed plans for extending the scale of Medicaid without always committing the federal government to pay the costs. In summer 2009, as the Senate Finance Committee (SFC) considered a Medicaid expansion on a federal-state cost-sharing basis, the National Governors Association wrote to the committee to protest: "Governors believe that reform of health care is critical to our nation's economic future. We also are steadfastly opposed to unfunded federal mandates and reforms that simply shift costs to states. The House has proposed providing permanent funding for its mandated Medicaid expansions. We urge your committee to adopt a similar approach for its bill."[15]

These anxieties crossed party lines, and Democratic governors—even those most sympathetic to comprehensive reform—urged their state senators to pressure SFC chair Max Baucus to bend.[16] In the end, he and his committee largely did so without conceding that the federal government would pay all costs down the line, and the Medicaid expansion became a reality in Title II of the ACA. At the time of the law's passage, the Congressional Budget Office (CBO) estimated 16 million Americans would get insurance as a consequence of the expansion.[17]

The importance of the expansion, however, lay not only in its scale but also in the way it reconfigured what might be termed the *values* underpinning the Medicaid program. Prior to the ACA, Medicaid and CHIP insured one out of every five Americans and included low-income seniors who had spent up their Medicare benefits, many Americans with severe disabilities, pregnant women, and children in low-income households. Nevertheless, in 2012, the program covered only 45 percent of nonelderly Americans living in households with an income below the FPL.[18] In short, a program routinely described as public health insurance for the poor did not even cover a majority of the nonelderly poor. In particular, reflecting long-standing value judgments about who is worthy of assistance, working-aged, able-bodied, childless adults were effectively excluded from eligibility in nearly all states. When Obama came into office, only five states allowed adults without children to enroll directly in Medicaid. The fact that the ACA proposed to impose a national minimum standard for Medicaid eligibility based solely on income-test criteria, without reference to "worthiness" or "responsibility," did therefore represent a profound philosophical shift.

In addition to expanding Medicaid, the framers of the ACA also set out to streamline the program's enrollment procedures, with an emphasis on getting state bureaucracies to reach out to vulnerable populations. Sections 2201 and 2202 of the ACA set out plans for a "single application for Medicaid, CHIP, and subsidized Marketplace coverage. All states must implement these simplifications, which are designed to better connect eligible people to coverage, regardless of whether they implement the expansion."[19] Although many states had turned to more "client-friendly" methods of enrollment throughout the 1990s and 2000s, "backsliding occurred at times, especially during recessions."[20] To reinforce the clauses of the ACA, in March 2012 the Centers for Medicare and Medicaid Services (CMS) issued a final rule stipulating that states would have to use an application process either determined by the secretary of Health and Human Services (HHS) or considered acceptable by the secretary. Furthermore, the "application must be available for individuals to submit online, by telephone, by mail, in person, and by fax and must be accessible to persons with limited English proficiency and people with disabilities at no cost to the individual. States may only request information that is necessary to make an eligibility determination."[21] One likely consequence of these simplified enrollment measures for state governments was that their Medicaid rolls would increase regardless of whether they opted into the wider ACA expansion through the so-called woodwork effect as people already eligible for, but not registered with, the state's pre-ACA program signed up for insurance coverage. Problematically for the states, the costs of providing coverage for these individuals would fall under the existing program funding mechanisms because such enrollees would not be *newly* eligible.[22]

POLICY LEGACIES, INSTITUTIONAL FRAGMENTATION, AND PUBLIC SENTIMENTS

Prior to the ACA's enactment, the Medicaid program had already embedded what might be termed *deep* policy legacies that weighed on policy makers as they contemplated how to react to new reform proposals for the program. This situation contrasted sharply with insurance exchanges, the ACA's other chief means of reducing numbers of uninsured, because the exchanges were to be new institutions with policy makers, therefore not influenced by feedback about how effectively they had worked in the past. Hence, analysis of how federal and state officials viewed the ACA's proposals with regard to Medicaid requires some examination of the insurance program's history in a manner not relevant to the policy design of the exchanges. This is particularly true because the policy legacies resulting from the prior evolution of Medicaid provided highly inconsistent feedback. Moreover, these inconsistencies were extensive, sending different messages to different actors and sometimes providing contradictory messages to the same actors.

Medicaid was established in 1965 as a program funded by a mix of federal and state dollars, with states having some discretion in terms of how extensive their funding, and hence the scope of their health provision through the program, would be. This funding arrangement contrasted with that of Medicare, organized and funded by the federal government, leading Medicaid to be perceived as the poor relation. Given its status as a means-tested program, it was commonly regarded as "welfare medicine." However, the program had built-in incentives for the states to spend their own money because the more a state spent, the greater the amount it received from the federal government. This led by 2001 to a situation where more spending through the program was "optional" rather than "mandatory" under the terms of federal regulations.[23] In fact, over time Medicaid belied its status as a "poor person's program" that would be politically vulnerable. Although significant cuts were made to the program in 1981 at the behest of the Reagan administration, in the later 1980s a series of incremental enhancements of the program expanded eligibility criteria.[24] Then, in 1997, the Clinton administration augmented it with the creation of CHIP, which provided health insurance to children in low-income families who did not qualify for Medicaid. The long-term expansionary dynamics of the program are illustrated by the fact that all fifty states increased their Medicaid spending in real terms, measured as spending on each person with income below the FPL, between 1992 and 2008.[25]

This story of the growing institutional resilience of Medicaid was not uniform across states. Conservative critics alleged that the incentive structure of the program was deliberately perverse. An American Enterprise Institute report alleged, "Medicaid is *designed* to be fiscally unsustainable—but politically self-sustaining." In the end, however, "something that cannot go on will eventually stop."[26] In short, according to conservatives, the funding scheme recklessly encouraged states to spend more of their own money to get more federal money. Whatever the merits of that argument, by the mid-2000s it was clear that for many states, Medicaid spending was crowding out other areas of important social spending.[27] In 2005, "reducing Medicaid expenses" was the "central item on the National Governors Association agenda," leading its members to call for significant restructuring of the program.[28] By fiscal year 2010, Medicaid spending accounted for 21.8 percent of state government expenditures.[29] Shortly before the Supreme Court's decision on the ACA in summer 2012, R. Andrew Allison, then president of the National Association of Medicaid Directors (NAMD), reflected that the "expansion of Medicaid is a sea change, and it's occurring at the most difficult fiscal time in the history of the program."[30] In fact states had long sought ways to contain their Medicaid expenses.

Thus, even as many states expanded their Medicaid eligibility and provision beyond the federal minimums, they simultaneously introduced measures that undermined the effectiveness of that provision. For example, a common practice was to cut payments to Medicaid providers. Even in 2010, thirty-nine states cut payments to providers.[31] Unsurprisingly, over time, this led many doctors to turn away new Medicaid patients.[32] In short, state officials were subject to a mixed array of policy feedback. On the positive side, if the state spent more of its own money, then it received extra federal dollars, allowing policy makers to offer more health care coverage to low-income households. On the downside, it was not always easy for states to fund their own commitments, and when they sought ways to contain costs, they risked limiting access to care for those very citizens they were trying to help.

Another important legacy in Medicaid was the increasing use of waivers granted by the federal government to the states that allowed states to diverge from federal rules and regulations. This phenomenon was given real momentum during the Clinton presidency.[33] In particular, after the failure of the Clinton reform effort in 1994, the number of statewide Medicaid demonstration projects authorized through waivers jumped in the mid-1990s, spiking once again in the mid-2000s.[34] Importantly, these waivers were not confined to small demonstration projects or research efforts designed by the federal government. As a Government Accountability Office (GAO) report noted, "States have used the flexibility granted through section 1115 to implement major changes to existing state Medicaid programs."[35] Many states, for example, used waiver authority to contract the treatment of some Medicaid recipients with managed-care organizations.[36] Consequently, by 2010 no two states had identical Medicaid rules and regulations.[37] As things stood in 2010, therefore, Medicaid was a program with uneven patterns of development between states and sometimes within states when expansion trajectories were reversed as a state's fiscal circumstances changed.[38]

As a result of the Supreme Court's decision in *NFIB v. Sebelius,* these policy legacies were accompanied by an institutional design for the Medicaid expansion marked by greater institutional fragmentation than the ACA's framers initially intended. As enacted, the ACA would have established a significantly higher national minimum standard of eligibility for the program and would have removed state discretion to make judgments about which categories of lower-income individuals were eligible for coverage. Hence, in institutional terms, the importance of the Supreme Court decision cannot be overstated. The decision undid the intent of the ACA's framers to establish Medicaid as, in effect, a new national entitlement program. The potentially game-changing nature of the ACA for the Medicaid program was in fact recognized in the Supreme Court judgment. Chief Justice John Roberts acknowledged that Congress had the authority to amend the Medicaid program but maintained that the ACA did not so much amend the existing Medicaid program as create a new one: "The Medicaid expansion . . . accomplishes a shift in kind, not merely degree. . . . It is no longer a program to care for the neediest among us but rather an element of a comprehensive national plan to provide universal health insurance coverage."[39]

In this context, the Court ruled that the sanctions the ACA imposed on states not complying with the expansion were too punitive.[40] The sanctions went beyond "encouragement," constituting a "gun to the head" because the states were not being given any realistic option to act autonomously.[41] The Court found the threat to withhold existing monies "coercive" and in the "opinion of the Court, federal co-ercion of states violated the core principle of federalism."[42] One important aspect of the Court's decision was the sheer scale of existing federal funding to the states through the Medicaid program. Roberts reflected on the importance of federal Medicaid dollars and noted, "The threatened loss of over 10 percent of a State's overall budget ... is economic dragooning," which meant that the states' theoretical choice of joining or not joining the expansion was not a choice at all.[43]

The immediate consequence of the Court's ruling was to allow fervent oppo-nents of the ACA at the state level to announce that they would not be expanding their existing Medicaid program. In institutional terms, however, the medium- to long-term impact of the ruling went beyond the rhetorical grandstanding because it reestablished the position of governors and state lawmakers at the center of the Medicaid decision-making process. The ACA had threatened to impose new rules on states in a manner that would have left many state officials disgruntled but effectively disempowered. Now, however, state actors were capable of dissenting, foregoing the promise of new federal transfers without losing existing Medicaid dollars. Yet, being presented with the opportunity to dissent was not necessarily a comfortable political position for some governors. It meant that the policy lega-cies discussed above, especially the contradiction between the temptation of extra federal dollars coming into the state versus anxiety about the long-term impact on state finances of committing to extra Medicaid spending, even on highly favorable terms, came back into view.

These pressures weighed heavily on the nation's governors. In comparison with the exchanges, which often required action by governors and legislatures to establish, the legacy of Medicaid had made governors the elected officials most associated with the decision about whether their states should expand their pro-grams, with the knowledge that if their states declined to participate there would be no alternative provision for those left uninsured, in contrast with the case of the exchanges. As holders of statewide office, they were also especially susceptible to pressures from hospitals and other medical providers who saw more Medicaid money as a means of reimbursement for what might otherwise be uncompensated care. In blue states with a history of generous Medicaid provision and a consensus to expand in line with the ACA, the choice was not as difficult for governors to make because they could participate in the expansion with the cooperation of the state legislature without regard to the Court's ruling. In deep red states with a past more skeptical of the value of liberal Medicaid eligibility, where the opposition to Obamacare was strong on the parts of both the governor and state lawmakers, in the short term at least, forceful dissent was a real option.

Elsewhere, however, cross-pressured governors, especially Republicans, faced more difficult choices.[44] The Court ruling did fragment authority for expanding the program, but it left in place the prospect of states receiving potentially billions of federal dollars, which made outright dissent more challenging. One way out of this dilemma for governors wishing to take the federal money but maintain some political distance from the ACA was to turn to the waiver process. The ACA in fact contained language suggesting an attempt to reduce the future importance of section 1115 waivers because it "specifically amended the Medicaid waiver process to ensure that it was used for genuine research, not political horse trading."[45] Section 10201(i) of the law required "public notice and comment, including public hearings, at the state level, and further public notice and comment at the federal level, before waiver programs can be approved and renewed."[46] In the institutional framework crafted by the Roberts Court, however, state governors now had leverage to persuade the federal government to allow them to experiment with alternative ways of expanding insurance to low-income households in their states through the well-established waiver process.[47]

The impact of public sentiments on the decisions of elected officials is difficult to gauge with any precision. As the public opinion data in Table 4.1 show, popular support for the Medicaid expansion was quite high overall, though attitudes were sharply divided along partisan lines. As the Kaiser Family Foundation's March 2013 tracking poll found, self-identified Democrats were strongly in favor of expansion, whereas a majority of Republican identifiers were opposed. Suggesting public sentiments were likely to have only a limited impact on decision making, the poll also found clear majorities of people did not know, at that point in time, what their state was doing with regard to the expansion, even when the state's governor had articulated a clear position.[48] Furthermore, although the forces in favor and against the expansion did create some unusual alliances among vested interests, debate about the specifics of the expansion was secondary to the ongoing bitter divide over the ACA as a whole. For most elected Republicans and identifiers, opposition to the ACA remained a touchstone at least until the 2012 election, and there was little attempt made in the public arena to tease out the separate elements of the reform for independent evaluation. As the expansion moved into clearer view throughout 2013 and came into force in 2014, there were signs the issue was developing increasing salience in nonexpansion states, with Democratic candidates sometimes attacking their Republican counterparts for their party's inaction.

The combination of longer legacies of federal-state cooperation, mixed institutional fragmentation, and partisan public sentiments suggests state-level opponents of the ACA faced a more complex environment when challenging the Medicaid expansion than in the case of the exchanges. As the following sections show, partisan challenges to the expansion could not always overcome the history of popular state efforts to expand Medicaid coverage and strong federal fiscal incentives to do the same.

Table 4.1 Public Opinion on Medicaid Expansion

Attitudes toward Medicaid Expansion, 2011–2013		
	Very or Somewhat Favorable	Very or Somewhat Unfavorable
November 2011	69%	26%
March 2012	70%	27%
April 2012	66%	32%
July 2012	67%	30%
March 2013	71%	27%
Attitudes toward Medicaid Expansion by Partisan Identification		
	Keep Medicaid as It Is Today	Expand Medicaid
Total	41%	52%
Democrats	20%	76%
Independents	46%	44%
Republicans	67%	26%

Source: Kaiser Family Foundation, Health Tracking Poll, March 2013, accessed November 14, 2014, http://kff.org/health-reform/poll-finding/march-2013-tracking-poll/.

NEGOTIATING CONSENT ON MEDICAID EXPANSION

From a federal perspective, initial planning for implementing the Medicaid expansion was based on the assumption that even reluctant states had little choice in the matter. As the ACA was debated in Congress, influential conservative think tank the Heritage Foundation issued a memo arguing that states would be better off withdrawing from Medicaid completely, and some states did investigate the possibility.[49] Nevada, for instance, commissioned a report to weigh the costs and benefits of opting out of Medicaid altogether. The resulting report noted, "Congress did not appear to envision a scenario where a state or states chose to act in their financial best interest by opting out of Medicaid."[50] The report itself did not come to a judgment over whether Nevada should opt out of Medicaid, but in listing the consequences of doing so for existing Medicaid beneficiaries, state agencies' and medical providers' rationale for staying in, even allowing for any extra burden to the state given the expansion, was compelling.[51] As Table 4.2 shows, the majority of states that did not ultimately adopt the Medicaid expansion engaged in similar studies. The Supreme Court decision, however, changed the fiscal calculation for states, giving the politics of dissent real meaning and the opponents of the ACA at the state level an opportunity to turn that dissent into substantive rejection of policy rather than symbolic protest against the federal government actions. In turn, this once again reinforced the importance of policy legacies, institutional arrangements, and public sentiments in the different states. For example, how much

Table 4.2 State-Generated Fiscal or Demographic Analysis of Medicaid
Expansion

	Publicly Available Program Analysis by State Agency	No Available State-Generated Analysis
States not expanding Medicaid	AK, FL, ID, IN, KS, LA, ME, MS, MT, NE, NH, OK, SC, SD, UT, WI, WY	AL, GA, MO, NC, TN, TX, VA
States expanding Medicaid	AR, AZ, CA, IA, KY, MD, MN, OH, PA, WA, WV	CO, CT, DE, HI, IL, MA, MI, ND, NJ, NM, NV, NY, OR, RI, VT

Source: State (Re)Forum, "Tracking Medicaid Expansion Decisions: A Closer Look at Legislative Activity," last updated February 7, 2014, accessed November 14, 2014, https://www.state reform.org/tracking-Medicaid-expansion-legislative-activity.

did it matter how generous pre-ACA Medicaid programs had been in a particular state? Furthermore, if institutions, notably governors and state legislatures, disagreed over expansion, where did power lie? How did public sentiments manifest themselves and influence behavior?

Initially White House aides downplayed the idea that the Supreme Court had opened the door to revolt against the expansion. On ABC's *This Week,* Obama's chief of staff, Jack Lew, said that the "vast majority" of states would still expand their programs, and "those few that are slow to come in, they're going to have to answer to people why they're turning this down and why they're letting people go without coverage."[52] In a more formal effort to contain any emerging dissent, Kathleen Sebelius, secretary of HHS, wrote to the nation's governors encouraging them to cooperate with the federal government in implementing the ACA. She thanked them for the "hard work" already undertaken in planning for the exchanges and then moved on to emphasize the financial gains that would accrue to states that proceeded with the Medicaid expansion. As part of the effort to persuade state authorities to work with the administration, her letter spelled out how enlarging Medicaid would benefit the medical industry in all states. Sebelius wrote that, despite the Court's decision, she was "hopeful that state leaders will take advantage of the opportunity provided to insure their poorest working families with the unusually generous federal resources while dramatically reducing the burden of uncompensated care on their hospitals and other health care providers."[53] Moreover, the projections of the amount states would need to spend to fund the expansion over the ten-year period from 2013 to 2022 contrasted significantly with the projected sums to be distributed by the federal government to the states. For example, Alabama would need to spend $1.081 billion over that period but would receive

$14.4 billion. Similarly, Georgia would spend $2.541 billion from its own budget in return for $33.3 billion from the federal budget, whereas Kansas would trade $525 million for $5.3 billion. By not joining the expansion these three states were forfeiting $7 billion, $12.8 billion, and $2.6 billion, respectively, in revenues to reimburse hospitals in their states.[54] These figures produced some unlikely allies for the administration. Craig Becker, president of the Tennessee Hospital Association, noted how in his state many local chambers of commerce had endorsed the principle of expansion: "These are rock-ribbed Republicans. . . . But they all scratch their heads and say, 'Well, if that's the case, then of course we do this.'"[55]

In fact, the explicit fiscal incentives and potential pressures from the medical industry did mean that more Republican governors oversaw Medicaid expansion in their states than supervised setting up health insurance exchanges. Sometimes they did this in collaboration with Democratic state legislatures. For instance, in Nevada, New Jersey, and New Mexico, the expansion was enacted without too much controversy. In other cases, however, Republican governors had to overcome fierce opposition from state legislatures controlled by their own party. In Ohio, for example, Governor John Kasich went to extraordinary lengths to bypass the state legislature. When the Ohio General Assembly made it clear that it would not cooperate with the governor's plans to opt in to the expansion, Kasich determined that a little known bureaucratic body in the state could authorize the expansion. Described in a *New York Times* report as an "obscure committee," the Controlling Board, "which normally oversees relatively small adjustments to the state budget," voted by a five-to-two margin to follow the governor's wishes.[56] When explaining his decision, Kasich emphasized that "we refused to run a state exchange," but the Medicaid expansion was a "chance to bring Ohio money back to Ohio to do some things that frankly needed to be done."[57]

Whereas governors such as Kasich and, as we will see below, Governor Brewer in Arizona had to battle to get the expansion implemented in their states, generally blue states with a history of relatively generous Medicaid provision embraced the expansion at the state level. This was the case even in states where existing Medicaid spending was putting a severe strain on the state budget. For example, Illinois was in negotiation with the federal government throughout 2012 to be allowed to toughen its eligibility requirements in the face of a looming budget deficit.[58] Yet, a year later, Democratic governor Pat Quinn signed the Medicaid expansion into law, which would add an estimated 342,000 to the state's Medicaid rolls. Quinn celebrated: "In the home state of President Obama, we believe access to quality health care is a fundamental right, and we proudly embrace the Affordable Care Act."[59] Similarly, in California, a state with a history of fiscal problems, the state government moved quickly to adopt the expansion.

A Case of Willing Consent: California

California provides an interesting case of a state government that embraced Medicaid expansion at the same time it was fighting sometimes acrimonious battles over health care policy with health care providers, labor unions, and the federal government.[60] In particular, the state was constantly trying to find ways to contain its own Medicaid spending, so as the debate progressed in Washington, DC, through 2009, the prospect of any new mandate to expand Medicaid not extensively funded by the federal government caused concern. In October 2009, Republican governor Arnold Schwarzenegger (2003–2011) voiced his support for a comprehensive overhaul of the US health care system but warned that any extension of insurance through Medicaid would have to be fully funded by the federal government. Otherwise, the "mandatory expansion will only be an empty promise of health insurance coverage and will force states like California to cut funding for education, public safety, or other important responsibilities."[61] In December 2009, in a letter to the California congressional delegation, he protested that leaving any of the cost of the Medicaid expansion to the states in the long term would constitute a "crushing new burden" that would "be added to a safety net that is already shredding under billions of dollars in unfunded federal mandates that we are struggling to meet."[62] Although Congress did not fully assuage Schwarzenegger's reservations about financing, he became the first Republican governor to endorse the ACA at the end of April 2010.[63]

Just two days before his announcement, Schwarzenegger had written to Secretary Sebelius reflecting on both the opportunities and challenges that implementing the ACA would bring to his state. In a letter cosigned by leading Democrats in the state legislature, Senator Pro Tem Darrell Steinberg (D-Sacramento) and Assembly Speaker John Perez (D-Los Angeles), the governor asked for leeway to amend the state's Medicaid program, known as Medi-Cal, and reflected, "The state's current fiscal situation poses another fundamental challenge as we begin the effort to implement national health reform."[64] Although emphasizing the state's fiscal predicament, however, the letter was also effectively asking for help in fast-tracking implementation of aspects of the Medicaid expansion and seeking to extend the use of managed-care plans for seniors and Medicaid beneficiaries with disabilities as a means of cost containment. In June, the California Department of Health Care Services applied for a waiver from the HHS, approved in November, to redesign the state program in order to curb spending growth and expand access.[65] The waiver application explicitly laid out how California could act as a model for the wider implementation of the ACA:

> California, with a population of 36.9 million, a Medicaid population of 7.5 million, and a burgeoning uninsured population of roughly 6.7 million is a perfect

microcosm to begin the long and complicated process of implementing national health care reform. Both the State's size and its diversity require that California, like the nation, begin to move steadily towards the coverage envisioned under the Patient Protection and Affordable Care Act (PPACA). Through a series of steps under a section 1115 waiver, California can lead the nation in articulating and resolving the inevitable issues that will present themselves as the State and nation move to implement the most sweeping social reform in 50 years.[66]

Under the terms of the waiver, California qualified for "$8 billion in federal Medicaid matching funds available for expanding coverage to low-income uninsured adults and preserving and improving the county-based safety net."[67] The money available from the federal government through the waiver reflected that, although full federal funding for the Medicaid expansion did not come until January 2014, the ACA stipulated that states could begin to enroll some of those newly eligible either through an ACA option or a waiver and would receive extra funding at their existing matching rate from the federal government.[68] In the end, California was one of five states, along with Connecticut, the District of Columbia, New Jersey, Minnesota, and Washington, that took the opportunity to begin the Medicaid expansion early.[69]

In late 2012 and early 2013, there were some tensions around how California would organize the full-scale expansion of Medicaid as Schwarzenegger's successor, Democratic governor Jerry Brown, negotiated with the state legislature and county officials about how the federal monies would be distributed.[70] In January 2013, Brown called for a special legislative session to deal with the difficulties in complying with the ACA. Brown spoke of the competing voices within the state administrative structures with regard to the Medicaid expansion: "Working out the right relationship with the counties will test our ingenuity and will not be achieved overnight," and with the "costs involved, great prudence should guide every step of the way."[71] In reality, however, there was little doubt that the state would press ahead with full expansion. In contrast to the implementation of the exchanges, during which insurers such as Anthem Blue Cross opposed the measures taken to comply with the ACA, there was no serious stakeholder opposition to the Medicaid expansion. One survey of lawmakers and health care stakeholders in the state found concerns about the potential strain on the state finances and worries about how effectively providing insurance would translate into providing actual care given the limited number of doctors accepting new Medicaid patients in the state; there was, however, general agreement on the value of pushing ahead with extending Medi-Cal coverage and on the importance of the Bridge to Reform waiver as a means of preparing the state for the full expansion.[72] The expansion also had the support of groups normally less sympathetic to the ACA; for example, the Los Angeles Area Chamber of Commerce supported the expansion as a means of reducing costs by diminishing the amount of uncompensated care.[73] Finally, in this supportive environment, in June 2013 the state legislature passed a budget bill incorporating the expansion signed into state law by Governor Brown. California's health and human services secretary, Diana Dooley, declared that expansion was something the "president made possible but we had to make real."[74]

Thus, despite the problematic policy legacies arising from the existing Medi-Cal program and the fact that the state had divided partisan government at the time of the ACA's passage, California became a pioneer in implementing the Medicaid expansion. As a blue state where, in contrast to the national numbers, opinion polls showed majority support for the ACA, it should not be especially surprising that California took the lead in implementing the new law in both Medicaid expansion and the health insurance exchanges, as suggested in the previous chapter.[75]

Arizona: A Governor Takes Control

Whereas California's expansion of Medicaid may have been taken for granted, the decision in Arizona to expand its Medicaid program was greeted with considerably more surprise. As *Politico* put it, it turned the state "into the unlikeliest of Obamacare allies."[76] In some immediate and obvious ways, that was true. Republican governor Brewer had been a formidable opponent to the Obama administration, especially over immigration policy, and had regularly denounced Obamacare. Moreover, the state legislature was in Republican hands, unlike those in neighboring Nevada and New Mexico, where Republican governors implemented the expansion. Yet some aspects of the previous development of Medicaid in Arizona should have provided a clue that the state might take the path it did. The state had in fact been one of the few to expand Medicaid coverage to childless adults up to 100 percent of the FPL prior to the ACA; significantly, that measure had been endorsed through a popular referendum. Thus, although the state cut back on its Medicaid enrollment in 2010 and 2011, advocates for expansion were able to portray the expansion as in line with the state's established policy trajectory.

Nevertheless, there was much conservative consternation and liberal surprise when Governor Brewer announced in January 2013 that she wanted the state to participate in the expansion. The surprise was a result not only of Brewer's previously solid conservative credentials but also her hostility to the ACA. As early as January 2009, in a move celebrated by ALEC, she ordered "state officials to abandon ObamaCare-related rulemaking."[77] When the governor announced her support for the expansion in January 2013 she described it as "one of the most difficult decisions" she had made but added that the state could not afford to miss out on the federal funding that would cover many of the state's uninsured and also bring health care jobs to the state. Before looking at events leading up to 2013, however, it is worth dwelling briefly on the state's rather contradictory previous relationship with the Medicaid program to understand how its institutional framework, policy legacies, and public sentiments toward the program affected developments.

Arizona was in fact the last state to sign up for Medicaid, only joining in 1982 and then only under the terms of a waiver granted by the Reagan administration allowing considerable flexibility in setting up the Arizona Health Care Cost Containment System (AHCCCS).[78] Yet, although initially a parsimonious latecomer to the program, the state did move to expand eligibility, including to childless adults. Moreover, that expansion of eligibility was confirmed through a state referendum. "Voters *twice* approved of extending AHCCCS coverage to childless adults with incomes at or below 100% FPL. In 1996, voters passed Proposition 203, Healthy Arizona I, with 72% of the vote."[79] That initiative, however, was not funded, but in 1998 the state received $3.2 billion over twenty-five years in an agreement with tobacco manufacturers. Then, using that as a funding source, in 2000 the voters approved Proposition 204, which again expanded coverage "up to 100% FPL by nearly 63% of the vote."[80] Furthermore, in 2002, voters "approved Proposition 303, a 60 cents per pack cigarette tax to help with the state's share of funding the AHCCCS expansion."[81]

Hence, Arizona quite quickly developed a relatively generous Medicaid program, at least if measured in terms of granting access to groups deemed ineligible in the vast majority of states. By the late 2000s, however, the state, suffering particularly from the collapse of the property market, had run into serious fiscal problems.[82] Conservative critics blamed Proposition 204 for these problems, particularly as the tobacco monies had not been enough to pay for the eligibility extension.[83] By 2010 Governor Brewer was proposing measures that would significantly eat away at the state's health care social safety net. In March 2010 she signed a budget that cut the state CHIP program, leaving 47,000 children potentially without access to insurance.[84] This was followed by a decision that the state would not fund certain organ transplants through Medicaid, though the backlash against that led to a policy reversal after six months.[85] Next, in January 2011, Arizona requested permission from the federal government to drop its commitments under Proposition 204 to insure childless adults up to 100 percent of the poverty line. This request was granted the following month by Secretary Sebelius, who noted that because the waiver under which Proposition 204 operated had expired in September 2011, it would not violate the clauses in the ACA stipulating that states could not reduce eligibility. It was estimated that this move would remove 250,000 adults from the state Medicaid rolls.[86]

Against this backdrop of consistent efforts to reduce the state Medicaid commitments, Brewer caused an uproar among conservatives when she advocated expansion in line with the ACA. An editorial in the *National Review Online* denounced her fiscal irresponsibility and denounced Medicaid as welfare spending.[87] A leading conservative think tank in the state, the Goldwater Institute, vigorously opposed the governor's initiative,[88] and the Arizona chapter of Americans for Prosperity quickly rebutted her rationale for the expansion.[89] Brewer tried to preempt this criticism by calling her decision the "conservative choice for Arizona." The governor's website further declared, "Nobody in Arizona has done more to oppose the Affordable Care Act than Governor Brewer." Interestingly, however, Brewer also framed the expansion as fulfilling the wishes of the Arizona citizens "who've twice voted to expand Medicaid."[90] State officials constantly invoked this latter point when they justified Brewer's new position. As reported in the *New York Times*, the Arizona director of Medicaid, Thomas Betlach, "refuses to use the word expansion. 'Restoration,' he said assertively during an interview, referring to the fact that under the governor's plan, the program would again apply to people who lost coverage when the recession hit and the state froze enrollment."[91] Brewer also received public support from health care workers and some business groups who emphasized the help the expansion would provide to the rural hospitals, which treated significant numbers of both Medicaid beneficiaries and people without insurance.[92] The health industry was particularly anxious to reverse the impact of the cuts to public health programs made in 2011. In the year after those cuts came into effect, some hospitals had "their budgets for uncompensated care quadruple," so hospital organizations lobbied hard in favor of the Medicaid expansion throughout 2012, at a time when Governor Brewer's office said she was undecided about how to proceed.[93]

Predictably, however, most of the Republican state lawmakers strongly opposed expansion. Arizona Senate president Andy Biggs declared that he would do "everything in my power" to stop the governor's plans.[94] The chances of expansion had, however, been improved by the results of the 2012 state legislative elections. The Republican Party still had majorities in both state chambers, but these had been reduced to margins of thirty-six to twenty-four in the House and seventeen to thirteen in the Senate.[95] This meant Brewer had to win over fewer members of her own party than would have been the case in 2012, but it was still a struggle. In late May 2013, frustrated by legislative inaction, the governor threatened to veto any legislation until action was taken; she made good on this promise on May 23, 2013, by vetoing five bills. Finally, in early June, "in a stunning political power play," Brewer called a special session of the legislature and, despite conservative Republicans making "hours of fiery floor speeches," there was sufficient bipartisan support to push the Medicaid expansion through the two chambers.[96]

Opponents, however, did not immediately give up. Promises of primary challenges were made to those Republican "Brewercrats" who had voted for "Obrewercare."[97] Furthermore, opponents sought to collect enough signatures to get a measure put on the state ballot that would have resulted in the expansion being frozen until November 2014.[98] In the end, the petition drive came up short, but opponents then turned to the courts, arguing that the law authorizing the expansion contained a new "tax" on hospitals rather than a new "fee." This difference in terminology mattered because Arizona law requires a legislative supermajority to raise taxes, and the expansion law had not been passed with such a majority.[99] By August 2014, after an initial victory for Governor Brewer but then a reprieve for the litigators, the Arizona Supreme Court agreed to take up the case.

The story in Arizona is complex and provides a narrative that does not fit easily with prevailing ideas about partisan behavior. It is instructive, however, to consider the significance of the policy legacies in the state. As governor, Brewer had sought ways of restricting and even reducing Arizona's Medicaid commitments, but its previous history of extending Medicaid coverage to some childless adults, endorsed through popular votes, did mean that expanding in line with the ACA could be framed as "restoring" the previous practice rather than doing something alien. In addition, the enrollment freezes put in place had a tangible impact on hospital revenues and thus meant that there was an energized constituency supportive of the expansion. Conservative opposition remained vigorous, but Republican majorities in the state legislature were not large enough to prevent a determined governor willing to work with Democrats to build a winning coalition.

CONTENTIOUS LEGACIES, INSTITUTIONAL FRAGMENTATION, AND THE POLITICS OF DISSENT

Clearly, the Supreme Court's decision on the ACA in June 2012 gave state officials the institutional capacity to meaningfully resist Medicaid expansion. Yet, even prior to that, high-profile Republican governors had complained about the prospect of implementing it. Importantly, whereas consent was constructed around the potentially huge influx of federal dollars to states to expand Medicaid and to reduce the number of uninsured, dissent resulted from *negative* policy legacies associated with the Medicaid program. In particular, governors and legislatures cited fiscal pressures caused by existing Medicaid spending, along with the likely extra costs states would incur as a consequence of both the "woodwork" effect and the long-term share of the cost of the expansion. In an article in the *Wall Street Journal* in early 2011, Republican governor Mitch Daniels of Indiana wrote,

> For state governments, the bill presents huge new costs, as we are required to enroll 15 million to 20 million more people in our Medicaid systems. In Indiana,

our independent actuaries have pegged the price to state taxpayers at $2.6 billion to $3 billion over the next 10 years. This is a huge burden for our state, and yet another incremental expenditure the law's authors declined to account for truthfully.[100]

Influential conservative voices also urged state officials to resist implementation of the expansion. Prior to the Supreme Court ruling, groups such as ALEC called on state lawmakers to consider completely opting out of Medicaid. The Heritage Foundation produced a study suggesting state governments would be better off outside the Medicaid program.[101] ALEC cited that report and advised state legislators, "Reframe the debate on Obamacare" to "introduce study bills or make public calls for Medicaid 'opt-out' in 2014 as a way to shift the debate to the unintended consequences of ObamaCare's Medicaid mandates."[102] As the ACA was crafted in Congress, some states—for example, Nevada, Texas, and Wyoming—did investigate whether they could save money by completely opting out of Medicaid, though none of them concluded that was a viable path.[103]

Empowered by the Supreme Court's decision, however, Bob McDonnell of Virginia, then chair of the Republican Governors Association, wrote to Secretary Sebelius making it clear he and many of his colleagues had significant reservations about expanding a program already stretching state budgets to the breaking point:

Even before increasing the Medicaid-eligible population as prescribed by PPACA, Medicaid has been on an unsustainable path, comprising [sic] a growing share of state budgets every year. It is difficult to see how expanding Medicaid without reform would do anything other than put more strain on state budgets and the taxpayers, especially when considering that many pernicious provisions that curtail state flexibility remain.[104]

Building on McDonnell's logic, Republican Mississippi governor Phil Bryant also provided a clear articulation of this perspective in spring 2013: "I continue to believe that Mississippi should not expand Medicaid because doing so would result in tax increases for hardworking Mississippians or cuts to critical spending in areas like education, public safety, and economic development."[105] In addition, the policy design of the ACA meant that the incentive structure for states with less generous Medicaid programs was double-edged. In parsimonious states, the pre-ACA programs left many individuals uninsured (who would have been covered in more generous states), so these states would have a relatively larger pool of *newly* eligible individuals attracting federal dollars. However, the temptation of those extra federal dollars was potentially offset by the fact that when the states did have to start picking up their share of the tab for the new beneficiaries, there would be a relatively larger number of new enrollees to subsidize.

Yet, as we have seen, decisions about Medicaid were less institutionally fragmented than the ones about the health insurance exchanges. The temptation of federal dollars did entice some Republican governors, and, as the examples of Arizona and Ohio illustrate, these governors exercised control on the issue. Wary of what it called "ObamaCare compliant governors," ALEC concentrated much of its attention on lobbying state legislators and urged them to ensure that governors could not act to implement any aspect of the ACA without the approval of their legislatures.[106] For example, in June 2013 the ALEC Legislative Board of Directors issued a model resolution for state legislatures to adopt that rejected the expansion.[107] Although governors did not always get their way, their positioning mostly determined the terms of the debate about expansion. Perhaps the single best example of the importance of the governor's identity for the fate of the Medicaid expansion came in the shape of Paul LePage in Maine, who took office in January 2011. The previous governor, Democrat John Baldacci, was committed to providing comprehensive coverage for everyone in the state. His efforts were thwarted by rising health care costs; his successor, the Republican LePage, moved in the opposite direction by cutting Medicaid eligibility.[108] LePage then repeatedly vetoed expansion plans passed by the Democratic legislature. Explaining one veto in April 2014, LePage referred to the cost of previous efforts to increase public insurance and maintained, "For the sake of the truly needy and Maine taxpayers, we cannot go down this path again."[109]

Public sentiments on the Medicaid program also mattered to these decisions. Because rejecting Medicaid expansion came at a clear cost to many of their citizens and to health care providers in the states, public officials justified their hostility using a variety of potent symbols. In addition to the concern about the impact on state budgets, some GOP governors expressed doubt that the federal government would maintain its commitment to pay 90 percent of costs in the long run. For example, in November 2013, just as the rollout of the health insurance exchange marketplaces seemed to be going awry, Governor Scott Walker of Wisconsin, a state with a history of relatively generous Medicaid provision, explained that he had "said no" to the expansion "because if I took the Medicaid expansion I'd be dependent on the same federal government that can't get a basic website up and going even after two and a half years to come through with payments for Medicaid in the future when they start weaning off paying for 100 percent of coverage."[110] Furthermore, many conservatives regard Medicaid as a broken system that ill serves both program beneficiaries and health care providers. They argue that adding millions more to the existing rolls will simply make matters worse.[111] Governor Perry, for instance, asserted that expanding the Medicaid rolls would be "like putting 1,000 more people on the Titanic when you knew what was going to happen."[112] Finally, some expressed their hostility to the principle of providing public insurance coverage to people who should be able to provide for themselves. In early December 2012, South Dakota governor Dennis Daugaard explained that, in his view, the potential new beneficiaries were not vulnerable people who needed public protection: "I want to stress that these are able-bodied adults. They're not disabled; we already cover the disabled. They're not children; we already cover children. These are adults—all of them."[113]

This list of concerns was always likely to persuade core Republican voters, but in addition, opponents sometimes framed dissent as a response to the federal refusal to make necessary changes to Medicaid. In particular, expansion opponents would often point to the problems with the existing Medicaid program and argue that before increasing the numbers on Medicaid it was necessary to fix those problems; fixing them, they claimed, would be best achieved by state governments, if only the federal authorities would give them the flexibility to go their own way. For example, in the 2014 gubernatorial battle in Texas, Democratic candidate Wendy Davis attacked her GOP rival, Greg Abbott, for his support of Governor Perry's rejection of the expansion. Abbott deflected the criticism by arguing that he wanted a waiver so that Texas could operate its Medicaid system under a block grant.[114] It was highly unlikely the federal government would accede to such a demand, but it provided a means for Abbot, like Perry before him, to deflect criticism of his actions onto a different target.

Unrepentant Opposition: Texas

As Chapter 3 suggested, if one person could be described as the poster child of opposition to the ACA, it would be Governor Perry. As the ACA passed Congress, Perry issued a press release saying the law was more about "expanding socialism on American soil" than solving the problems of the country's health care system. The statement concluded, "Texas leaders will continue to do everything in our power to fight this federal excess and find ways to protect our families, taxpayers, and medical providers from this gross federal overreach."[115] At that time, it was not clear what capacity the state had to resist the ACA, and throughout summer 2010, despite Perry's rhetoric, state bureaucrats, including then state Medicaid director Billy Millwee, began preparing for the ACA rollout.[116] Toward the end of the year, after the November 2010 elections had reinforced Republican control of the state, a number of conservative lawmakers did begin to talk of a complete Medicaid opt out, and the governor also raised this possibility.[117] The legislature commissioned a report by the Texas Health and Human Services Commission to investigate the impact of such a move. As with similar investigations in Nevada and Wyoming, the report detailed the manner in which this would lead to a significant increase in the number of uninsured in the state and how hospitals in particular would be burdened with providing even more uncompensated care.[118]

Although the idea of opting out of Medicaid was quietly dropped, state officials did put forward waiver requests asking for greater flexibility in running the program, including choosing which services to provide in the state.[119] Underpinning these requests was the worry about a looming fiscal deficit in the state, but the flexibility Secretary Sebelius had indicated she was prepared to allow states in terms of tightening eligibility did not have much application in Texas because the state did not offer much in the first place in the way of optional extras through its Medicaid program. The limited nature of the Texas Medicaid program reflected the fact that prior to the ACA, the state had been one of the least generous (or, depending on the perspective, most prudent) of states in terms of its Medicaid eligibility for its adult population. Medicaid and CHIP did cover 3.6 million Texans, but the state did not offer any coverage to childless adults of working age without disabilities, and it covered parents of dependent children to only 12 percent of the FPL for those who were jobless and 25 percent for those with work. Only Alabama and Louisiana had stricter eligibility measures on both these counts.[120] Despite the frugality of the state provision, however, Medicaid spending still accounted for a significant share of overall state expenditures. When explaining Perry's sympathy for the idea of withdrawing from Medicaid, a spokesperson complained that Medicaid consumed 20 percent of the state budget.[121]

Hence, the policy legacies of Medicaid in Texas offered few positive signals for supporters of health care reform. In the context of the state budget, the program was expensive, yet the level of provision did not prevent the state from having the highest rate of uninsured in the nation, with 24 percent of the state population lacking health insurance in 2012.[122] Whereas the expansion anticipated by the ACA's framers in 2010 would have significantly reduced the number of uninsured, when the Supreme Court made the expansion voluntary, the Texas political leadership focused on the former legacy and the cost to the state of maintaining its existing Medicaid spending, not to mention increasing it. Thus, although the Urban Institute estimated that over ten years Texas would receive $65.6 billion in federal funds while incurring a cost of $5.7 billion if it opted in to the expansion, Governor Perry and a united Republican state establishment rejected that choice.[123] Days after the Supreme Court decision, Perry wrote a letter to Secretary Sebelius summarizing his objections to the ACA. With regard to Medicaid he noted, "Through its proposed expansion of Medicaid, the PPACA would simply enlarge a broken system that is already financially unsustainable. Medicaid is a system of inflexible mandates, one-size-fits-all requirements, and wasteful, bureaucratic inefficiencies. Expanding it as the PPACA provides would only exacerbate the failure of the current system, and would threaten even Texas with financial ruin."[124]

Texas Democrats protested, and organizations such as Texas Well and Healthy brought together coalitions of proexpansion advocates.[125] Their arguments were bolstered by opinion poll evidence suggesting that most Texans did favor expanding the Medicaid program when that option was put to them as an independent question.[126] Furthermore, reflecting how some business groups normally allied with the Republican Party disagreed with those opposed to the Medicaid expansion, the chambers of commerce representing some of the largest Texas cities, including Arlington, Dallas, Fort Worth, and San Antonio, lobbied in favor of it. The chief executive of the El Paso Chamber of Commerce, Richard Dayoub, reflected, "This may be the only time that we have taken an actual formal position that is opposite that of the governor." He added, "I don't know of any issue that has created so much concern across the state and has amassed so much support across party lines and throughout the business sector."[127] However, no GOP state lawmakers announced public support for the expansion, and, whatever the support for the specific idea of Medicaid expansion, the ACA as a whole remained unpopular in the state.[128] In summer 2013, Governor Perry reiterated his opposition to the expansion. Responding to the fact that more than 1 million Texans would gain Medicaid coverage under the terms of the Medicaid expansion, the governor stated, "Texas will not be held hostage by the Obama administration's attempt to force us into this fool's errand of adding more than a million Texans to a broken system."[129]

A Governor Rebuffed: Florida

Like Texas, Florida stood aside when the Medicaid expansion took effect in January 2014. Yet, like Arizona, it had a Republican governor who had surprised the state's political elites by coming out in early 2013 in support of the expansion. Unlike Brewer, and unlike Kasich in Ohio, however, Governor Scott was unable to achieve his aims because the Republican-controlled state legislature would not be bypassed and refused to authorize the expansion. In fact, Scott had been an even more unlikely convert to the merits of the expansion than Brewer had. Both had presented themselves as staunch opponents of the ACA, but Scott had been much more explicit in his objections to Medicaid expansion than Brewer had ever publicly been. At the time of the ACA's passage, Florida's governor was Charlie Crist (2007–2011). Crist was also a Republican but willing to work with the Obama White House. Interestingly in light of future developments, the state legislature rebuked the Crist administration in October 2010 for proceeding with ACA implementation without its authorization.[130] When Scott, who had made opposition to the ACA central to his political image from the very start of his campaign for the GOP nomination, replaced Crist in 2011, it seemed the new governor was going to be more in tune with the Republican leadership in the state legislature than his predecessor was.[131]

Scott reinforced this image after Judge Roger Vinson's ruling in federal district court in Pensacola, Florida, declared the ACA unconstitutional. In response to Vinson's ruling, Scott announced that state agencies would not work to implement the law until "we know exactly what is going to happen," adding, "and I hope and I believe that either it will be declared unconstitutional or it will be repealed."[132] Furthermore, after the 2012 Supreme Court ruling, Scott was even quicker to the draw than Perry in announcing his state would not participate in the expansion. Although more than 20 percent of Florida residents lacked insurance at the time, Scott said Medicaid was already undermining state fiscal stability because the program costs were "growing three and a half times as fast as Florida's general revenue," and the long-term cost for the state related to its share of funding the expansion would be too much of a burden for the taxpayers.[133] Like other figures justifying dissent, Scott referred to policy legacies associated with the cost of the existing state Medicaid commitments to explain that the state could not afford the expansion.

As a result, there was considerable surprise and anger in conservative circles when Scott switched his position on the merits of Medicaid expansion in early 2013. He explained his change of heart by saying, "I cannot, in good conscience, deny Floridians access to health care" when the costs are being borne by the federal government.[134] Although Scott talked of maintaining the expansion only through the opening three years when the federal government would bear all the cost of insuring the newly eligible, the projections over ten years illustrated the scale of funding the state would potentially receive if it opted in over the long term; Florida would need to spend an estimated $5.36 billion before 2022, with more than $66 billion in federal funding coming into the state to insure more than 1 million Floridians. The gap between estimated potential federal funds and potential long-term state expenditures was the largest of that of any of the states that had not expanded their programs by 2014.[135] Despite these numbers, however, and illustrating the importance of institutional fragmentation at the state level, the state legislature did not support Governor Scott. Furthermore, and unlike in Arizona, where Governor Brewer strong-armed the state lawmakers, or Ohio, where Governor Kasich bypassed them, Scott did not use the power of the executive branch to push his plans through. A particularly powerful foe was House Speaker Will Weatherford, and his chamber effectively ruled out any compromise. Although the House rejected Scott's requests, the Senate was prepared to contemplate taking the federal money as long as beneficiaries were enrolled in private insurance plans rather than Medicaid; but led by Weatherford, the House rejected the entire prospect of a federally funded expansion.[136] Weatherford, who got billing as one of the rising stars of the conservative movement at the 2013 Conservative Political Action

Committee conference, told that gathering, "They're trying to buy us off, one by one, but I am not buying it. . . . Florida will not buy it, and America should not buy it. We will stand up to their inflexible plan, and we'll work on our own solution, one that better reflects the needs and priorities of our state. Here's the bottom line: It's time for the states to take a stand."[137]

Scott's position in favor of expansion had been reinforced by the endorsement, if in guarded language, of two major business organizations, the Florida Chamber of Commerce and Associated Industries of Florida.[138] This did not persuade the Republican majorities in the state legislature, and Scott chose not to engage in the type of institutional brinksmanship Brewer used. Democrats urged Scott to threaten to veto the state budget unless Republican legislators cooperated, but he chose not to exercise executive power in that way. One factor working against any such move was the size of the GOP majority in the House, which at the start of 2013 stood at seventy-four to forty-six, meaning that Scott would have needed to get a large number to break ranks from Weatherford's leadership. Additionally, the fact that Scott had previously agitated against the expansion, calling it unaffordable, provided grounds for continued opposition from conservative lawmakers. Moreover, Florida had little in its historical record to suggest that it would look enthusiastically at a dramatic extension of Medicaid eligibility because the state had "long ranked relatively low on indicators of Medicaid effort, falling into the bottom quartile of states on both expenditures and enrollees per poor person."[139] As with Texas, some public opinion polling suggested a majority of Floridians supported the expansion, yet the nature of the determined opposition in the state legislature coupled with the state's laggard history with regard to Medicaid, meant that Governor Scott's tepid leadership was unlikely to prevail.[140]

HYBRID REFORMS

One effect of the Supreme Court's decision in *NFIB v. Sebelius* was to empower state governments in their negotiations with the federal authorities over the Medicaid expansion. As the Obama administration accepted the possibility of seeing many millions of the uninsured remain uninsured in nonexpansion states, there was now an incentive for policy makers at HHS to bargain and accept that some states would do expansion in their own distinctive fashion. By May 2014, six governors had asked for waivers, meaning that their states would receive the federal expansion dollars but would be able to diverge from the terms of the expansion as laid out in the ACA. Five of these governors were Republicans, including Governor Mike Pence of Indiana, who remained steadfastly opposed to his state setting up its own exchange and who, as a member of Congress prior to becoming governor, had voted on numerous occasions to repeal the ACA.[141] Governor Pence demanded that Indiana be allowed to enact the expansion through the Health Indiana Plan (HIP). By virtue of a section 1115 waiver granted by the George W. Bush administration, through HIP, Indiana had used "Medicaid funds to provide a benefit package modeled after a high-deductible health plan and health savings account to previously uninsured very poor and low-income adults" since January 2008.[142] This was a controversial waiver when it was granted, given the Democrats' long-standing distaste for health savings accounts, so the negotiations between the Pence and Obama administrations on the extended use of this model as a means of expanding the state Medicaid program continued delicately during 2014.[143] In fact, the White House demonstrated in August 2014 that it would not concede too much ground to the states. That moment came when the Republican governor Tom Corbett of Pennsylvania successfully negotiated some concessions, allowing that state to diverge from the ACA, but Corbett's plan "tying Medicaid eligibility to employment, requiring enrollees to either be working or actively job searching," was rejected.[144]

Although the Pennsylvania example shows the limits of bargaining, the Obama administration had reached out to "persuadable" red states to get them to engage with Medicaid expansion on amended terms. In particular, HHS officials sent out signals that the department would look favorably on waivers seeking to use subsidized private insurance to cover low-income households. According to a spokesperson for HHS, "Our goal in working with states has been to be as flexible as possible within the confines of the law."[145] In early 2013, as the private insurance option gained traction because of initiatives in Arkansas and Ohio, Matt Salo, then director of the NAMD, noted that these states would provide a model for others: "If Arkansas and Ohio can find a path through this thicket, it could give a lot of other states that have either said 'No' or are on the fence a reason to think again."[146] Arkansas in particular was a leader in negotiating an alternative version of the expansion.

The Third Way: Arkansas

At first glance it might seem odd that Arkansas would be a state even considering opting in to the Medicaid expansion. Before ACA's implementation, the state had some of the most restrictive eligibility requirements for adults in the nation and offered no coverage to childless adults.[147] Furthermore, despite this relative parsimony, there was concern about the burden of continuing Medicaid spending borne by the state even before any costs associated with expansion kicked in. For Arkansas, the extra costs of implementing Medicaid expansion were projected to be relatively higher than for almost all other states. One early simulation found that if all states achieved the 57 percent participation rate among newly eligible enroll-ees anticipated by the CBO, then Arkansas would see its own Medicaid spending increase by 4.7 percent between 2014 and 2019 from a baseline assuming that the ACA had not been enacted, compared with an average of 1.4 percent across all the states.[148] Yet state officials did not display the hostility to the Medicaid expansion seen elsewhere in the South, and the state did not join the lawsuit against the ACA. In summer 2012, then Arkansas surgeon general Joseph Thompson welcomed the "huge opportunity" the Medicaid expansion offered "to provide coverage for low-income citizens that we simply cannot afford without federal financing."[149] At that point in time, unusually for a southern state, Arkansas had unified Democratic government, with Governor Mike Beebe a supporter of expansion.

Importantly, however, the partisan balance in the state changed significantly between the enactment of the ACA in spring 2010 and the time for the final state decision making in 2013. After controlling the state government by comfortable margins, the Democrats were reduced to small majorities in the 2010 elections, and, in 2012, the GOP took control of both the House and Senate for the first time since the 1870s.[150] Yet, rather than follow the example of their counterparts in Flor-ida and rebuff a governor seeking to implement the expansion, the GOP majorities in the Arkansas state legislature initiated discussions to find an alternative path that would simultaneously bring the federal funding to the state, cover the popula-tion targeted by the ACA's Medicaid plans, and be acceptable to conservatives.[151] This last aspect did mean that a straightforward expansion of Medicaid was not on the agenda, but the willingness to craft a deal brought positive responses from both Governor Beebe and the federal government.

In essence the proposal was to use federal Medicaid dollars to provide private insurance to working-aged adults using a qualified health plan available through the health insurance exchange. This so-called private option built on the "premium assistance" authority already embedded in Medicaid, if little used, which allowed states to buy private insurance using Medicaid funds as long as that insurance was no more expensive than traditional Medicaid.[152] This last requirement did raise some concerns because the CBO had suggested in 2012 that private insurance cost 50 percent more than Medicaid, but in March 2013 the Arkansas Department of Human Services reported that its proposed model would result in minimal extra costs at worst.[153] As the plans were developed, the state received verbal agreement from Secretary Sebelius that they would be approved.[154] The plans were formalized in the Health Care Independence Act (HCIA), which passed both chambers of the state legislature by the three-fourths margins required in the state for an appro-priations measure.[155] In August 2013, Governor Beebe officially put forward a sec-tion 1115 demonstration waiver request. In his letter to Sebelius, Beebe concluded, "We appreciate the assistance your department has offered and look forward to your continued support."[156] The following month, the waiver was approved, leading Beebe to comment, "Arkansas came up with its own plan to expand Medicaid using the private insurance market, and Secretary Sebelius and her team worked to ensure that we had the flexibility to make that plan a reality."[157]

Whereas Governor Beebe expressed his pleasure at the outcome and the fact that more than 200,000 Arkansans would be newly eligible for insurance, the Republican architects of the HCIA were anxious to present their plan as one of dissent rather than as a compromise equivalent to negotiated consent. For example, as the plan was being developed, Republican state senator Jonathan Dismang insisted, "A lot of people would like to say this is moving the football down the field. In fact, what I think we've done is intercepted, and we're taking the ball in the other direction."[158] Later, as the law took effect, he maintained that the private option fundamentally changed the nature of the Medicaid program: "By employing conservative principles, the Arkansas act dismantles the traditional Medicaid structure and specifically addresses identified shortcomings. Despite popular national opinion that we would be unsuccessful in our negotiations, to date, the state has effectively leveraged its position to make unprecedented steps toward true entitlement reform."[159]

Other conservative voices, however, were less convinced. Nicole Kaeding, policy manager of the Arkansas chapter of Americans for Prosperity, lamented, "The Arkansas Scheme is just expansion by another name."[160] Nina Owcharenko of the Heritage Foundation was no more impressed, describing the Arkansas plan as "private coverage in name only."[161] These criticisms, from implacable foes of the ACA, were predictable, but the conservative backlash against developments in the state briefly seemed to upend the private option expansion in early 2014. Whereas the federal government granted a three-year waiver to Arkansas, the HCIA needed annual reauthorization by a three-fourths majority in both chambers of the state legislature. When the measure came up in February 2014, it seemed as if it might fall a few crucial votes short in the House. In 2013, the law had garnered 77 votes out of 100, evidence that about half the Republican delegation was prepared to support the private option expansion. Yet, given the state institutional requirement to have an annual vote that reached a three-fourths majority, it also showed that the coalition underpinning the HCIA was fragile. In these circumstances, each vote became critical, and tensions rose in February 2014 as the vote for reauthorization neared and conservatives promised primary challenges to those GOP lawmakers who had supported the law in 2013. In the end, it took five counts in the House before the 75 votes needed were achieved, and this only came with some amendments from conservative dissenters who openly acknowledged their desire for the expansion effort to fail. Most notably, the reauthorization bill dictated that state funds could not be used to promote outreach efforts to encourage people to sign up for the program.[162]

Overall, as in Arizona and Florida, the events in Arkansas need careful unraveling to understand the outcomes. In Arkansas, the policy legacies might seem to militate against expansion, but, importantly, the state government was under the control of Democrats until 2012—and the governor, the state director of Medicaid, and other leading state officials were supportive of expansion in order to significantly reduce the legacy of uninsured in the state. The governor's role was critical in continuing to work with Republicans after that party took control of the state legislature, and by early 2013 the federal government had displayed willingness to discuss alternative ways of providing health insurance coverage to the target population. For their part, those Republicans who took the lead in negotiating the private option were able to frame their plans as distinctive from, and even opposite to, the expansion as outlined in the ACA.

CONCLUSION

In its original form, the ACA would have fundamentally changed the nature of the Medicaid program, effectively making it an entitlement for people living in households with incomes under 138 percent of the FPL. The effectiveness with which states implemented the new rules would have varied according to their political willingness to accommodate the reforms and their administrative capacity to do so, and, given the unwillingness of some doctors to treat Medicaid patients, the fact of having coverage would not automatically have translated into easy access to care for beneficiaries. Yet, unless a state had taken the dramatic decision to drop Medicaid entirely, then each state would have had to comply with the ACA, however grudgingly.

By striking down the capacity of the federal government to sanction states that did not comply with the Medicaid expansion, the Supreme Court significantly rewrote the institutional design of the ACA. Now, rather than access to Medicaid becoming an entitlement for individuals in low-income households, it remains dependent on each state's policy makers. State policy makers could still embrace the huge fiscal incentives and engage with the expansion on the terms and conditions laid out in the ACA, but they could also express their dissent in a meaningful manner and, despite pressure from powerful interests such as hospitals, refuse to participate in the expansion. In addition, the option of renegotiating the terms and conditions of engagement became an option for states, and the early months of 2014 suggested that developing ways of using public money to insure poorer households via private insurers was the most likely way in which more states would participate over time.

This divergent reaction to the expansion after it became voluntary should not have come as a surprise. First, regarding policy legacies since the 1990s, Medicaid waivers had led to a plethora of different practices in the states. Although some policy issues were common across all states—notably, the pressure to simultaneously increase their own spending in order to receive more federal revenue yet to restrain that spending to prevent Medicaid costs crowding out other important aspects of the state budget—policy makers could emphasize different aspects of those legacies in order to justify their response to the ACA. Positive legacies of popular coverage expansions could be used to justify further enlargement of the program, as we saw in the case of Arizona. In states such as Texas, Medicaid had a more negative legacy for consuming a large chunk of the state's budget while leaving many uninsured. These negative legacies acted as constraints on expansion.

Second, the fragmented institutional logic of the Medicaid expansion allowed entrepreneurial governors to set the agenda, with large fiscal transfers as incentives. As the examples of Arizona and Florida show, a governor could fight more or less aggressively to get his or her way. This is not to argue that Governor Scott in Florida could have prevailed against the wishes of the state legislature, but he did not demonstrate the zeal of Governors Brewer and Kasich, who stretched their executive authority to the limit.

A final piece of the jigsaw is public sentiments. Here, the story suggests that the partisan framing of Medicaid as part of "Obamacare" constrained expansion. Polls show that, even in deep red states such as Texas, there is majority support for the expansion if it is framed as an independent issue, but the public was rarely exposed to sustained debate about individual elements of the ACA in this fashion. Moreover, although the issue gained salience among party activists, especially in the GOP, in which primary challengers for state legislative elections attempted to use votes about expansion as political weapons, the public, especially the potential beneficiaries of the expansion, remained poorly informed.

5. Regulatory Reform: The Quiet Politics of Bargaining and Consent

To expand access to low-cost health care, the Patient Protection and Affordable Care Act (ACA) does not rely solely on the Medicaid expansion or the broadened availability of tax subsidies for the purchase of care on health insurance exchanges. Complementing these efforts, the ACA contains a suite of regulatory reforms requiring that insurance providers improve transparency in the cost of their services; provide reasonable justifications for premium rate hikes; and cap the portion of premiums they can spend on profits, sales expenses, and administrative costs as opposed to medical claims and improvements in the quality of care.[1] However pivotal to the ACA, the politics of these regulatory reforms differs critically from health insurance exchanges and Medicaid expansion; unlike the reforms we have reviewed thus far, it has been challenging for opponents to foster widespread state refusals to cooperate with regulatory reforms. As these reforms rolled out, Republican governors did not launch vocal campaigns of resistance; states did not generally directly refuse to cooperate with these provisions; and organized interests opposed to these reforms, such as insurance companies, have not yet engaged in vituperative rhetoric over what they perceive as the illegitimacy or unconstitutionality of the reforms. Although Republican governors and legislatures were never especially sanguine about the ACA's regulatory reforms, partisan control of state governments does not get us especially far in explaining the patterns of postreform politics we describe in this chapter. Though states had varying regulatory regimes for the health insurance market prior to ACA's passage, most states gave their insurance commissioners basic authority to monitor premiums and to protect consumers. Furthermore, regulators at the state and federal level interpreted the ACA's reforms as not requiring extensive additional legislative action at the state level to comply. This allowed state regulators to implement reforms under their existing authority and removed the veto points to state participation that had existed in the case of the exchanges and the Medicaid expansion. Partisan opponents in the legislatures wishing to engage in dissent now had to build a coalition to undermine existing state policies, an obstacle most could not surmount. Finally, the low salience of regulatory reforms, especially compared with other parts of the law, made it difficult for opponents of the ACA's regulatory reforms to generate the energy necessary to undermine the regulatory changes brought on by health care reform.

The near absence of the dissent pattern described in Chapters 3 and 4 does not mean, however, that state-level opponents *endorsed* the ACA's regulatory reforms. After the law's passage, and especially after the 2010 midterm elections, conservative policy organizations such as the American Legislative Exchange Council (ALEC) targeted the ACA's regulatory reforms for reversal, as seen in Chapter 2. Insurance industry groups such as America's Health Insurance Plans (AHIP) also remained bitterly opposed to stringent interpretations of the medical loss ratio (MLR), which they have repeatedly criticized for limiting what health plan providers can spend on a "variety of programs and services that improve the quality and safety of patient care" and which prevent the industry from undertaking innovations that will ultimately benefit consumers.[2] Insurance companies have also publicly disagreed with decisions of federal and state regulators to declare their premium rate increases "unreasonable," insisting rate hikes are based on rising costs and increasing use of medical services.[3] Some have declared that they will proceed with premium increases regardless of regulatory decisions.[4]

Nevertheless, organized opposition to the ACA did not result in the kind of state actions we described in the previous two chapters. Republican state legislatures did not prove to be the sites of resistance to regulatory reform that ideological opponents had hoped. Their attempts at killing regulatory reform through legislation largely failed. Though the insurance industry had different motivations and goals than Republicans and ideological conservatives, it pursued an "inside strategy" that relied on influencing debates between insurance commissioners and federal regulators about the substance of the reforms. As one industry observer put it in 2012, "Insurers are not going to be out there saying, 'Repeal, repeal, repeal.' . . . They will probably try to find the particular provisions that cause them heartburn, but not throw the baby out with the bath water."[5]

This chapter shows that opponents of the ACA faced three challenges in constructing dissent. First, regulatory reform in the ACA emerged from a long legacy of state-level engagement in market regulation, supported by state insurance commissioners. Facing pressure from partisan and ideological opponents of the ACA, state and federal regulators bargained over the minimum standards of the ACA's "early market reforms" so that states did not have to enact any new legislation or regulations in order to participate. Rather, insurance commissioners in most states could act under their *existing authority* to implement the law. Similarly, state insurance regulators bargained with federal officials to produce minimal rate review regulations that required little additional positive action beyond what was already "on the books." With the MLR, a preexisting legacy of state regulatory action drew opponents to intergovernmental bargaining rather than noisy legislative politics. In each of these cases, preexisting policy legacies fostered the negotiation of consent.

Second, the low level of institutional fragmentation in the ACA's regulatory reforms gave opponents little opportunity to engage in dissent. Because the Department of Health and Human Services (HHS) quickly set minimum standards on rate review and early market reforms that state governments could adopt with little or no additional legislative action, opponents of these reforms wishing to engage in dissent would have had to build new legislative coalitions to gut the existing authority of insurance commissioners. Thus, in contrast to the exchanges or Medicaid expansion, the veto points in the state legislative process stacked the deck against opponents rather than working in their favor. The MLR was more streamlined still. Though the ACA required intergovernmental bargaining over MLR rules, it enabled HHS to impose the rules emerging from bargaining and to decide whether states could receive waivers to exempt them from the new requirements, a structure that further preempted dissent legislation within the states.

Finally, although opponents theoretically could have promoted dissent by bringing regulatory issues into focus in state legislatures, public sentiments made this challenging. Compared with the exchanges, which directed consequences on consumer behavior, and the symbolically weighty Medicaid expansion, regulatory reforms were exceptionally complex and difficult for the public to appreciate, especially because they had a more immediate effect on the behavior of producers rather than consumers. Moreover, opponents seeking to sow public dissent may have had a difficult time converting regulatory reforms into recognizable objects of public scorn. Taken together, these factors provided incentives for opponents to use intergovernmental bargaining as the means to contest the ACA's regulatory reforms.

To begin, we briefly illustrate the core policy issues involved in the ACA's regulatory reforms. We then discuss the three features of the reforms (legacy, institutional design, and public sentiments) that made it especially difficult for opponents to engage in the construction of dissent. Third, we show how opponents engaged in the negotiation of consent through the processes of consultation, rulemaking, and waiver bargaining. Fourth, we illustrate the difficulties opponents faced in engaging in dissent relative to regulatory reforms. We conclude by discussing the results of these processes of negotiation, which will continue to shape the ACA as it develops over time and across state contexts.

POLICY ISSUES

There are numerous regulatory reforms within the ACA, ranging from enhanced standards for the kinds of coverage plan information insurance companies must provide to consumers to prohibitions on companies' denial of coverage because of preexisting conditions.[6] As Chapter 2 revealed, the law's regulatory provisions rolled out in waves. During the first year, federal and state regulators implemented so-called early market reforms designed to *expand access to care*. These provisions included prohibitions on denying coverage because of preexisting conditions and worker salaries, requirements that insurance plans cover dependents until age twenty-six, and expansions of the scope of care that plans must provide across insurance markets, large and small.[7] These early market reforms mirrored some provisions in the Health Insurance Portability and Accountability Act of 1996 (HIPAA). HIPAA took incremental steps to expand access to care in a number of ways, including limiting insurers' ability to exclude individuals from coverage based on preexisting conditions and requiring that insurers offer small-group health plans to small employers. To accomplish these goals, HIPAA required that states ensure that their health insurance laws conformed to new federal rules.[8] The ACA's early market reforms, sometimes called the "patient's bill of rights," were built on HIPAA's framework and rolled out in September 2010.[9]

In addition to reforms that expanded access to coverage, the ACA contained provisions designed to lower the cost of care. The reform included stronger standards for reviewing premium rate increases by insurers. Rate review is the process by which insurance regulators review the new or renewed rates for health plan insurance policies, ensuring that the rates charged are based on accurate, verifiable data and realistic projections of health care costs.[10] Although state insurance departments have managed rate review in the past, these practices have varied in stringency.[11] Most importantly, a number of states lacked legal authority or resources to review rates prior to their implementation. Under the rules promulgated by HHS in accordance with the ACA, annual rate increases of 10 percent or more must be reviewed for their reasonableness prior to their implementation, and insurers must also publicly justify rate increases.[12] If a state rate review program meets the new minimum federal standards and is deemed an "effective rate review program," HHS will accept the state determination of whether such rate increases are reasonable. If the state rate review program does not meet the minimum federal standards, federal regulators will conduct reviews of rate increases of 10 percent or more to assess their "reasonability."[13]

Though the ACA's statutory provisions for rate review contain some specific details, Congress left the development of the review process to the secretary of Health and Human Services, who worked in conjunction with state insurance commissioners at the National Association of Insurance Commissioners (NAIC).[14] In particular, the secretary was directed to work with states to develop minimum standards for effective rate review by which states must abide, including both the kind of rate data states must collect from insurance companies and the process through which they must analyze this data. Additionally, states were directed to work with the secretary to define what counts as an "unreasonable" rate increase. Finally, the states may apply for grants from the secretary to improve their rate review processes.

The ACA also regulates the way insurers use the premiums they collect in order to provide better value to consumers. To make this happen, Congress focused on regulating insurers' MLRs. The MLR, used even before the ACA passed, is an assessment technique used by state regulators, insurance companies, and investors to measure the percentage of premium dollars collected from policyholders that contributes directly to paying for care versus what goes to overhead and profits.[15] Traditionally, if an insurer had a 75 percent MLR, it spent 75 percent of premium dollars directly on insurance claims and 25 percent on expenses that did not contribute to claims. However, during debate over the ACA, these kinds of expenses, including "executive pay, advertising costs, agent commissions, and profits," came under serious congressional scrutiny as contributors to the ballooning cost of care.[16]

Under the ACA, Congress created an MLR regulation applicable to most insurance companies that covered individuals and small businesses. The ACA's regulatory provisions include both specific statutory mandates and provisions up to the interpretation of the secretary of Health and Human Services, working in collaboration with state insurance regulators.[17] Congress specifically mandated that insurance plans, both in the individual and small-group markets, attain an 80 percent MLR and that large-group plans attain an MLR of 85 percent. In addition, Congress required insurance companies to release data on premium revenue. Furthermore, companies that do not meet the ACA's minimum MLR requirements must provide an appropriate rebate to consumers.[18] Although it created significant numerical cutoffs, Congress also adjusted the formula for the MLR. Whereas the majority of the insurers' MLR was once calculated by dividing premium dollars spent on health care claims by the total number of premium dollars, the ACA allows insurers to include some nonclaim expenses toward calculating the 80 percent minimum. It also adjusts the denominator of the ratio by subtracting premium dollars spent on federal, state, and local taxes and regulatory licenses and fees.

Yet when Congress designed the ACA's MLR provisions, its members did not clearly specify what counted as "quality improvement expenses." Instead, it directed HHS to consult with the NAIC in developing uniform definitions of expense categories and standardized methodologies and calculating them.[19] After these regulations were finalized, HHS alone, not the states, was to enforce them. Even so, the ACA permits HHS to waive MLR numerical cutoffs whenever state insurance commissioners provide a reasonable justification, based on the characteristics of their state insurance markets, to do so.[20] The effectiveness of the MLR in delivering consumer value as well as its direct monetary effect on insurance companies' bottom line depends on the expenses insurance companies can and cannot count as contributions to the quality of health care. As the number of expenses insurers can claim as essential to quality improvement expands, the benefit to consumers shrinks, and vice versa. Unsurprisingly, then, the intergovernmental debate over these provisions became crucial in the rollout of the MLR provisions.

POLICY LEGACIES, INSTITUTIONAL FRAGMENTATION, AND PUBLIC SENTIMENTS

The policy context for implementing the ACA's regulatory reforms differed from that of exchanges and the Medicaid expansion in that state implementation required less positive action, especially when it came to the enactment of new legislation or regulations (see the summary in Table 5.1). First, regulatory reforms in the ACA built upon preexisting frameworks that gave state regulators authority to carry out policies without extensive additional authorization from state legislatures. Although only Massachusetts had created a prototype health insurance marketplace prior to the ACA's passage, states overall tended to be much more familiar with regulatory reforms. In 1980, states and their insurance regulators attempted to synthesize stronger, more harmonized health insurance. Still, the states' regulation of insurance markets began even earlier than that in response to the 1869 Supreme Court ruling in *Paul v. Virginia* that insurance regulation fell squarely within the authority of states.[21] Thereafter, an emergent field of state insurance commissioners formed the National Insurance Convention, now known as the NAIC.

The NAIC's organizational development contributed substantially to the persistent decentralization of insurance regulation in the United States. Though the Supreme Court later ruled in *United States v. South-Eastern Underwriters Association* (1944) that federal insurance regulation was constitutional under the commerce clause authority of Congress, Congress passed the McCarran-Ferguson Act one year later, which exempted most forms of insurance from federal regulation, leaving the task to states.[22] Between 1945 and the present, the NAIC continued to coordinate regulation between states and generate norms in the field of state insurance regulation. In 1980, the NAIC expanded its policy work to the health insurance market, publishing the *Guidelines for Filing of Rates for Individual Health Insurance Forms*.[23] These guidelines, which have come to dominate the field of state insurance regulation, grew out of a process of bargaining between regulators, industry groups, and consumers at the state level, rather than through sharply partisan debates.[24] The NAIC's decision rules reflect this logic; the association typi-

Table 5.1 Regulatory Reform Policy Contexts

	Early Market Reforms	Rate Review	Medical Loss Ratio
Policy legacy before ACA	38 states had basic authority on access and rating guarantees; 12 states had HIPAA "federal fallback" standards	47 states had some rate review provisions for the individual market	34 states required insurers to report MLR; 27 had specific ratio requirement
Institutional fragmentation	Decision making: HHS set federal minimum standards implementation: federal preemption if states did not meet minimum	Decision making: HHS defined minimum standards, in consultation with NAIC implementation: federal preemption if states did not meet minimum	Decision making: HHS consulted with NAIC to define "quality improvement expenses" and other terms; direct federal enforcement implementation: direct federal enforcement, with state-requested adjustments
Public sentiments	Salience: high support: high	Salience: low support: unclear	Salience: low support: high

cally delegates important decisions to small committees made up of experts and representatives of industry and consumers. Such decisions are rarely overturned when the NAIC meets in full session, and partisan politics tends to be subordinated to cooperation and bargaining.[25]

The NAIC's efforts at harmonization did not create uniformly *robust* regulations across the fifty states but did help states to create regulatory frameworks upon which Congress eventually built when it passed HIPAA. As Table 5.1 shows, prior to the ACA, thirty-eight states had their own standards designed to broaden access to coverage in the individual market. Most states also possessed statutory authority on rate review. All fifty states had laws on the books giving insurance regulators some form of authority to examine insurers' premium rate increases and the insurance plans they sold. These varied in strength. Twenty-six states had the authority to reject rate increases before they went into effect. Other states could only review premium increases or issue determinations retroactively (so-called file-and-use provisions after the rate was already in effect).[26] Similarly, thirty-four states allowed regulators to review insurers' MLRs, and twenty-seven imposed specific MLR standards on insurers.[27] As with rate review, these standards varied across states. Prior to the ACA's implementation, New Jersey set 80 percent MLR requirements, and some states such as North Dakota set an especially low bar of 55 percent.[28] Despite the uneven strength of these policies, most state regulators had the flexibility to widen their scope of authority without further legislative authorization. Even regulators in states such as Alaska and Utah, who operated under a minimal file-and-use statute, were able to use their authority to negotiate more modest rate increases with insurers.[29]

The ACA's rate review and early market reform provisions further minimized the need for state legislatures or governors to take positive action by not setting specific and high goals states would have to meet in order to comply. Rather, Congress required officials at the newly created Office for Consumer Information and Insurance Oversight (OCIIO), initially led by former Missouri insurance commissioner Jay Angoff, to negotiate with the NAIC in setting minimum federal standards.[30] To insulate OCIIO from political challenges, the Obama administration reorganized it in early 2011 as the Center for Consumer Information and Insurance Oversight (CCIIO) and placed it under the control of the Centers for Medicare and Medicaid Services (CMS).[31] Both Angoff and his 2011 replacement, former Maryland insurance commissioner Steve Larsen, bargained with state regulators over what states had to do to comply with early market reforms and to establish "effective" rate review programs, a term Congress did not define in the legislation. When HHS determined that a state rate review program was ineffective or out of compliance with market reforms, federal officials were allowed to step in.[32] Yet unlike the states, permitted to go even further to prohibit unreasonable rate increases above 10 percent, HHS could only review increases, make determinations about their reasonableness, and make public announcements about unreasonable increases.[33]

Although MLR reforms allow for intergovernmental negotiation and state regulatory waivers from federal standards, they go a step further in minimizing states' need to take positive action by requiring direct federal implementation.[34] Legislatures and governors might involve themselves with MLR reform but only to establish parallel regulatory systems that exceed the "floor" established by the law.[35] Additionally, both rate review and MLR reform streamline federal enforcement. In this regard, MLR contains sharper "teeth" than rate review. In the event HHS can identify industry noncompliance with MLR provisions, Congress granted the department freedom to impose monetary penalties on responsible parties directly, without the involvement of state governments.[36] All of these features suggest opponents had greater opportunities to shape the ACA's regulatory reforms during intergovernmental bargaining than in legislative battles.

A final distinctive feature of the policy context for the ACA's regulatory reforms is the climate of public opinion, marked by low salience and public approval

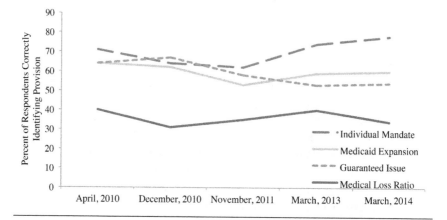

Figure 5.1 Public Knowledge about Select ACA Provisions

Source: Kaiser Family Foundation, Health Tracking Poll, March 2014, accessed October 24, 2014, http://kff.org/health-reform/poll-finding/kaiser-health-tracking-poll-march-2014/.

for regulatory reforms. In summer 2012 as the MLR, rate review, and other regulatory provisions were going into effect, elite opinion leaders had remarkably little to say about them, and coverage remained limited to boutique publications. Major media outlets chose to focus instead on the bill's more controversial provisions, especially the individual mandate, the subject of the landmark *National Federation of Independent Business (NFIB) v. Sebelius* case in the Supreme Court.[37]

Public opinion polls reflected greater support for regulatory reforms than for Medicaid expansion and the individual mandate, which opponents criticized in tandem with health insurance exchanges. In February 2012, for instance, the Kaiser Family Foundation's tracking poll revealed broad public support for the ACA's regulatory provisions, especially consumer protections.[38] Yet unlike with Medicaid expansion, which opponents latched onto as a symbol of reckless spending, the ACA's regulatory provisions were of much lower salience. As Figure 5.1 shows, public opinion polls that asked respondents to correctly identify the ACA's provisions revealed that 27 percent of those surveyed in April 2010 were less likely to correctly identify the content of the MLR reforms as a part of the ACA. The twin patterns of public support and low salience are perhaps unsurprising considering that concentrated producer groups are most likely to be adversely affected by regulatory reform, whereas diffuse health consumers stand to benefit. Additionally, because regulatory reform is conceptually complex, it may also be difficult for insurers to mobilize the kind of symbolic politics of "welfare" or "big government" mobilized in response to the ACA's other major reforms.[39] Together, then, these data points would lead us to believe the public was not mobilized to react negatively to the ACA's regulatory reforms, making the dissent strategy difficult for opponents to engage in even if the institutional architecture of the reforms had been more amenable.

The context for implementing the ACA's regulatory reforms appears to have been primed for the politics of consent and bargaining. State-level policy legacies, though not uniformly indicative of a strong regulatory regime, may have signaled the ACA's opponents that state legislatures were not viable venues for launching a high-intensity critique of regulatory reforms because this would require repealing preexisting laws. Similarly, the institutional design of the ACA's regulatory reform provisions appears to have effectively limited opponents' opportunities to engage in dissent by minimizing the need for positive action by governors and legislatures and crafting stronger enforcement provisions in the case of the MLR. Finally, public sentiments appear not to have been propitious for advocates of dissent. Without an especially mobilized opinion on regulatory reform, dissent may not have worked even if opponents had the opportunity to engage in it seriously. In the sections that follow, we provide more systematic evidence that links the policy context to the politics of regulatory policy.

THE NEGOTIATION OF CONSENT

Although the politics of the ACA's regulatory reforms may have been quiet, it was nonetheless fraught with confrontation. In the face of a tough political environment for reform, HHS officials such as Angoff and Larsen—led by the White House—were quick to bargain with states, ratcheting down requirements for states to enact new legislation or develop new regulations to come into compliance with the act. Yet in contrast to the reforms we described in previous chapters, bargaining—not dissent—persisted even after the Republican sweep of state offices in 2010. In this section, we review broad patterns in the negotiation of consent across three regulatory reforms and then illustrate these patterns by focusing on implementation efforts in Connecticut and Indiana.

Early Market Reforms:
The White House and the Manufacture of Success

In 2010, the White House was on "red alert" regarding the implementation of the ACA's early reforms to the insurance market. For political strategists at the White House Office of Health Reform (OHR), including its director, Nancy-Ann Min

DeParle, the first priority was to avoid a collision course with states where opposition to the ACA was strong. For those like Angoff at OCIIO, this meant a fair share of tongue biting as White House strategists such as DeParle negotiated with governors and state insurance regulators over the reform. As one source told us, the agency "didn't breathe" without White House approval.[40]

Whereas OCIIO had initially interpreted the early market reforms as requiring extensive proof that states had taken action to revise their market rules, informal OHR consultations with governors and state insurance regulators revealed this to be too politically fraught. Republican-dominated states declared that they did not intend to pass new reforms. Confidential spreadsheets tabulating state efforts to change their individual market policies were, as a federal official put it, "mostly red," meaning that a majority of states had refused to take action.[41] Had regulators required states to pass new laws or enact new regulations to comply with the ten early market reforms, around half of the states would have been deemed "out of compliance."

Yet after bargaining with state officials over the summer, DeParle's OHR used the ACA's statutory ambiguity and the fact that most states had regulatory frameworks for the individual market to, as one state regulator put it, "bend over backwards" for the states.[42] Eager to avoid the image of a policy blunder in which states refused to pass new legislation, the White House insisted that OCIIO adopt a new, minimal standard. As long as states issued subregulatory guidance or indicated that they were reviewing insurance policies, they would be considered to have "substantially enforced" the law. Noncompliance turned into compliance "overnight"; red spreadsheets suddenly became green.[43] Although five states (Alabama, Missouri, Oklahoma, Texas, and Wyoming) ultimately refused to take action on reforms, most states responded positively to this deal by the time new state governments took office in 2011. Republican strongholds were overwhelmingly likely to have done the minimum to remain compliant (see Table 5.2).

The effectiveness of these minimal compliance standards remains unmeasured. Federal efforts at data collection on state implementation of reforms slowly withered after the 2010 elections. OCIIO, and later CCIIO, had little interest in developing a reputation for "parachuting" into states and inspecting their regulatory procedures. Rather than "command-and-control" enforcement, the strategy was to rely on consumer-generated complaints.[44] At least one state regulator reported that the absence of federal pressure to create new regulations or legislation would allow them to effect policy change more quietly, without pressure from the governor or state legislature.[45] Nevertheless, the absence of extensive state action requirements preempted the high-profile state legislative challenges that occurred in the cases of Medicaid expansion and the exchanges.

Table 5.2 State Action on Early Market Reforms, 2010–2011

	State Partisan Composition after 2010 Elections	
	Unified Republican Government	Unified Democratic Government, Divided Government, or Other
Passed law or issued regulation on all ten reforms	IN, ND, SD, VA	CT, HI, IA, MA, ME, MD, MN, NC, NE, NY, OR, VT
Passed law or issued new regulation on at least one market reform	UT, WI	AK, CA, CO, DE, IL, LA, NH, NJ, NV, RI, WA
Issued subregulatory guidance on all ten reforms	GA, MI, PA, SC	AR, KY, MT, NM
Conducted form review on all ten reforms	AZ, FL, ID, KS, MS,# OH, TN	WV
Took no action	AL,* OK, TX,* WY	MO*

*Regulator initially reported cooperation but later retracted. State partisan control refers to the date when grant funds were returned. Partisan control in Iowa, Kansas, Louisiana, Mississippi, New Jersey, New Mexico, South Carolina, and Virginia reflects 2011 off-cycle or special election results.

#Republicans only took full control of the Mississippi legislature after the November 2011 state elections.

Source: Katie Keith and Kevin Lucia, *Implementing the Affordable Care Act: The State of the States*, Commonwealth Fund Brief (New York: Commonwealth Fund, 2014), 13.

Rate Review: The Floor Stays Low

Although the process of negotiating rate review regulations took longer than early market reforms and involved longer NAIC negotiations, it unfolded in a similar way, with state regulators negotiating more flexible federal standards in a climate of state-level opposition. In April 2010, HHS issued a call for comments to aid in the development of rate review regulations.[46] Federal regulators were particularly interested in the procedures states already had in place to review premium rates and rate increases. Which categories of cost increases did states find permissible? What kinds of data did states use to calculate costs? Finally, what kinds of cost information did states require insurers to disclose?[47] The NAIC's answers to these questions would help to solidify a low floor for rate review provisions—partially disabling opponents' attempts at preventing federal-state cooperation.

Within a month, the NAIC had assembled its Executive Committee to issue a response to HHS that began to put flesh on what exactly the term *unreasonable rate increase* might mean. AHIP, an organization of insurance industry lobbyists, urged the NAIC to adopt a particularly weak standard based on such factors as an insurer's ability to pay the cost of estimated claims. Insurers also insisted more elaborate standards made no sense and might be capriciously applied by regulators.[48] However, when the NAIC responded to the HHS request for information, it avoided advocating any particular definition of the word *reasonable*. Instead, its letter included eleven possible approaches to defining unreasonable rate increases, including but not limited to increases based on incorrect actuarial data (an idea suggested by AHIP), increases over a particular numerical cutoff or higher than the Consumer Price Index (CPI), and increases that resulted from excessive administrative expenses or profits.[49] As one NAIC member put it, "We didn't think it would be reasonable to have a discussion on whether X is 2 percent or 10 percent or 30 percent, but to say, here are the alternatives."[50] To the chagrin of AHIP and consumer groups alike, the comments refused to endorse one standard, emphasizing the variability of preexisting state policies as well as the fact that most state regulators attempted to balance rate review techniques, such as auditing and reporting, to provide consumer protection while avoiding unnecessarily severe penalties on insurers.[51]

When the NAIC concluded its 2010 session, it did not recommend that state insurance commissioners be authorized to reject unreasonable rate increases, nor did it recommend that HHS abide by uniform rate review procedures set by federal officials.[52] Additionally, along the lines of its response to HHS, the NAIC urged federal officials to keep the standard for reviewing rate increases flexible enough to meet the multiple justifications insurers might have for increases. Beyond that, the NAIC rejected the term *unreasonable* in favor of the phrase *potentially unreasonable* to describe rate increases.[53] These decisions suggest that though intergovernmental bargaining did not guarantee insurers their preferred regulatory agenda, the NAIC remained a site where their influence had demonstrable and, from their perspective, often positive results.

When HHS published its final rate review rule in 2011, it generally followed the recommendations outlined by the NAIC, preempting future legislative challenges in the states. First, HHS did not establish nationwide criteria for what counted as an "unreasonable rate increase," allowing states to rely on their preexisting statutes and regulations to define this term. Under the proposed rule, states were permitted to apply their own standards for determining what counted as a reasonable justification for a rate increase.[54] Because the language of the entire rule hinged on whether rate increases above 10 percent were reasonable, this was especially consequential. HHS established its own standards for defining unreasonable increases, such as excessiveness (increases that resulted in a projected future loss ratio below the federal MLR), lack of substantial evidence or appropriate assumptions, and unfairly discriminatory differences in premiums for consumers with similar risk categories. Although these criteria were on the strong side, they applied only in states that did not possess effective rate review programs as determined by HHS.[55]

Though the department ultimately allowed states to define what counted as an unreasonable increase, it did put into place minimum criteria states had to meet before they were permitted to conduct their own independent rate reviews. In addition to requiring states to construct a statutory or regulatory definition of reasonableness, HHS crafted four standards from common review practices, summarized in the NAIC's communications to the agency. First, state insurance departments had to have written procedures for determining whether rate increases were reasonable according to state-based standards. Second, HHS required states to have a procedure for reviewing data provided by insurers about proposed rate increases. Third, states were required to independently examine whether the assumptions made by the insurer proposing an increase were "reasonable" using thirteen specific kinds of data, including major trends in medical costs.[56] Finally, the proposed regulation required that states have a regulation or statute on the books clearly defining what was or was not reasonable.[57] In cases in which states did not meet minimum requirements, HHS would have the authority to review rate increases but not to reject them in accordance with the ACA's language. Nevertheless, HHS emphasized that as long as a state "can conduct an effective review of proposed rate increases that meet or exceed the applicable threshold," HHS would not "second-guess" them by conducting its own review.[58] Similarly, HHS crafted a nationally applicable rule to trigger reviews of premium increases of 10 percent or more but indicated that state-specific thresholds would be desirable if states could provide sufficient data to show that they were warranted.[59] These regulations would remain in place when HHS published the final rule in 2011. By the time it had finished rulemaking in 2011, forty-two states were deemed to have "effective rate review" programs. Within the next three years, an additional three states would bring their policies into line via subregulatory guidance, regulation, or minor legislative adjustments.[60] By 2014, only five states lacked effective rate review programs. These were, as it happens, the same five states that ultimately refused to enforce the early market reforms—Alabama, Missouri, Oklahoma, Texas, and Wyoming. As our discussion of the politics of dissent will suggest, this limited number of exceptional states demonstrates just how difficult it was for opponents to mount a coherent legislative challenge to the ACA's regulatory reforms.

Medical Loss Ratio: Bargaining under the Watchful Eye of Congress

As with rate review, negotiations over the MLR featured intense clashes between supporters and opponents of new regulations. However, MLR rules did not ignite a firestorm of state legislative challenges. Unlike in the last two examples, the process that generated this outcome did not result in lower federal standards. Rather, because the ACA allowed for direct federal implementation of the reform, state opposition to stronger federal standards was inconsequential. Combined with vocal congressional opposition to weak MLR standards, direct federal implementation weakened the bargaining power of states where opposition was strong.

In spring 2010, long before the HHS-proposed regulations were released, the NAIC set up working groups of state insurance commissioners to analyze and make recommendations on MLR provisions.[61] One group focused on developing a form for reporting MLR components, and another developed categories of expenditures permissible as "quality improvement activities," counting toward the 80 percent MLR set by Congress.[62] At the outset, insurers and consumer groups wrangled over insurers' definition of "quality improvement," which consumer representatives believed could allow insurers to reclassify administrative expenses as contributing to health quality.[63] Consumers and insurers also debated how HHS should calculate insurers' MLR. Whereas insurers claimed MLR data should be aggregated at the national level, consumers believed this would create a loophole in which insurers could violate the MLR rule in some states without having to pay rebates as long as their *overall* MLR exceeded the 80 percent threshold. Consumer representatives thus proposed that insurers' MLRs should be calculated for each state individually.[64]

Although opponents of tougher market regulations actively participated in discussions on both the MLR and rate review, their influence on the NAIC's decisions about the MLR differed for at least one important reason: the watchful eye of Senator Jay Rockefeller (D-WV). Rockefeller had been the architect of MLR reform in the ACA and became its advocate in the NAIC's deliberations.[65] In addition to providing explicit committee reports to accompany the legislation to spell out the specific intent of Congress with the new standard, Rockefeller closely watched the NAIC's deliberations. When he became concerned that insurers were attempting to covertly retrench MLR reforms by influencing state regulators to adopt relaxed standards, Rockefeller brought the issue up in letters to HHS secretary Kathleen Sebelius and NAIC president Jane Cline, again emphasizing that the intent of the MLR legislation was clearly to ensure "most of consumers' health insurance premiums dollars should pay for patient care, not for insurers' administrative costs and profits."[66] Such clear intent, he suggested, militated against national aggregation of data and broad interpretations of terms such as *quality improvement*.[67]

Rockefeller wasted little time responding to industry pressure on the NAIC. In July 2010, he counted that insurers had submitted 160 letters to commissioners, totaling 600 pages in length, compared with 23 letters submitted by consumer representatives. Incensed, he wrote a public letter to Cline describing in detail how insurance companies were trying to "game" the reform against the public interest.[68] Cline defended the association's work, but the NAIC was without a doubt "on notice" and responded by narrowing its definition of quality improvements, insisting that they, at a minimum, be based on evidence, be capable of objective measurement, and advance the delivery of patient-centered care.[69] When insurers pushed for revisions to these definitions in October 2010, Rockefeller struck back again, insisting that the NAIC forbid insurers from "spoil[ing]" its work.[70] With this kind of pressure, the NAIC sent its recommendations to HHS without substantial industry revisions in late October.[71]

Negotiations over the HHS interim final rule (IFR) on the MLR, published December 1, 2010, differed substantially from those held on rate review. First, because the IFR incorporated the NAIC's more stringent recommendations in full, insurers continued to debate the rule's classification of quality improvement expenses.[72] Insurers and other interest groups continued to argue that the IFR's definition of quality improvement expenses was too narrow and would prohibit insurers from pursuing innovative techniques to improve the quality of care. Consumer advocates and health care providers pushed back, suggesting that an overly broad interpretation of the congressional language would nullify the purpose of MLR reform.

Second, even when insurers were more successful at negotiating with the NAIC, the ACA's provision for direct federal implementation undercut state regulators' bargaining power. A case in point here is the HHS decision about agent and broker fees. As published, the IFR calculated fees paid to agents and brokers as administrative costs rather than quality improvement expenses because these fees did not lead to direct improvements in the quality of care or direct spending on claims.[73] Consumer advocates and the American Medical Association (AMA) supported this rule, arguing that agent and broker fees were "quintessential administrative costs."[74] Insurers, health underwriters, agents, and brokers all sent comments to HHS opposing this rule.[75] The US Chamber of Commerce joined in, arguing, "Agents and brokers serve a critical role in the health care marketplace, aiding consumers and employers in determining the health plan that best suits their needs at a premium they can afford."[76]

At first, the NAIC did not take an opposing position on the rule because it had been a proponent of the reform in its initial recommendation to HHS. Yet the 2010 elections changed the composition of the NAIC, bringing in additional commissioners from Republican states where opposition to the ACA ran high.[77] This revived the NAIC's interest in collaborating with insurers to oppose the IFR's agent and broker provisions. Leading the effort was Florida insurance commissioner and NAIC president-elect Kevin McCarty.[78] In March 2011, McCarty led a task force to develop recommendations to exclude agent and broker commissions from the MLR calculation.[79] Again, Rockefeller stepped into the fray, writing to members of the NAIC that these efforts would undermine the legislative intent of the MLR. Rockefeller's letter was part of the material distributed at the NAIC's spring meeting, where members considered McCarty's recommendation.[80] In May, Rockefeller's Commerce Committee report showed that removing agent and broker commissions from the MLR calculation would result in reduced rebates to consumers by more than 60 percent, totaling $1.1 billion.[81] This data evidently gave the NAIC's membership some pause, and in July, in response to opposition from several members, the organization temporarily shelved McCarty's proposal.[82] However, by November, McCarty presented a slightly modified version, urging HHS to both exempt agent and broker commissions from the MLR calculation and place a hold on MLR implementation in order for state waiver requests to be filed, rather than endorse the proposed legislation in full.[83] The resolution passed twenty-six to twenty over strong objections from some members of the NAIC. As Sandy Praeger, a commissioner from Kansas, put it: "We [the NAIC] were written into the [ACA] because we were trusted as experts on this. We are going so far here as to put our credibility in jeopardy."[84]

For all the bluster, McCarty's effort amounted to nothing. On December 7, 2011, HHS finalized its MLR rule (CMS-9998-FC) but made only the minor modifications that MLR reform opponents had requested.[85] For instance, it refused to permit fraud reduction expenses to count as quality improvement measures, as insurers had advocated. Those modifications HHS did make concerned more minor issues, such as shifts in how the rule would calculate quality improvement expenditures for smaller health plans.[86] Similarly, subsequent amendments to the rule made between 2011 and 2012 lacked major adjustments.[87] Because the law did not give the states significant implementation authority, opponents of the MLR would continue to bargain with individual state regulators.

In 2011, a study by the Government Accountability Office (GAO) found that insurers were adjusting brokers' fees and other costs in order to comply with the MLR.[88] However, this did not signal the end of their engagement with intergovernmental bargaining. Rather, they worked within the boundaries of the MLR to negotiate their consent. In particular, insurers and right-leaning ideological interest groups such as Americans for Tax Reform urged states to request waivers for the MLR 80 percent requirement, claiming that the high standard would cost jobs, disrupt markets, and cause higher premiums.[89] As Figure 5.2 shows, even in states where opposition to the ACA was particularly robust, intergovernmental bargaining became a primary mode of challenging the ACA.

The case of Texas provides insight into how the waiver process worked in a state steadfastly opposed to the ACA. Under pressure from insurers, the Texas Department of Insurance (TDI) requested an MLR waiver. TDI commissioner Mike Geeslin used the waiver to criticize the ACA, arguing that the MLR 80 percent

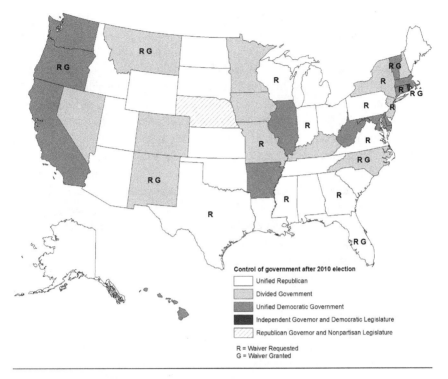

Figure 5.2 State Medical Loss Ratio Waiver Requests and Approvals

Note: Partisan control in Iowa, Kansas, Louisiana, Mississippi, New Jersey, New Mexico, South Carolina, and Virginia reflects 2011 off-cycle or special-election results.

Source: Kaiser Family Foundation, *Medical Loss Ratio Adjustments,* http://kff.org/health-reform /state-indicator/medical-loss-ratio-adjustments/. Partisan control data compiled by authors from Ballotpedia.com.

requirement in the individual insurance market would "stifle competition in the market and constrain many Texans' access to coverage."[90] TDI proposed to roll out the change slowly, starting at 71 percent/29 percent in 2011 and increasing the ratio by 3 percent each year until it reached 80/20 in 2014.[91] Yet the political mobilization around the waiver went further. In addition to the Texas application package, HHS received twelve public comments, including two letters from Texas legislators and its congressional delegation as well as a petition signed by 2,775 Texans opposing the 80 percent standard.[92] Supporters of the rule also engaged in the discussion; eleven public interest groups opposed the department application, arguing that it was unnecessary and that honoring it would lead to rising premiums.[93]

HHS ultimately denied the Texas request, claiming primarily, "Texas laws provide little incentive for issuers to exit before the individual market reforms take hold in 2014."[94] In particular, HHS showed that thirty issuers included in the TDI application remained in the market, and eleven of those met the 80 percent MLR standard or were very close to meeting it. Of the issuers who would not meet the 80 percent, three issuers have changed their pricing models to reach an 80 percent standard. The Texas concerns over market exit were thus largely overstated. Among other reasons it cited for denying the Texas application, HHS claimed that the TDI had not adequately shown consumer access to agents and brokers would be adversely affected by the 80 percent MLR standard.[95] In response to the denial of its application, the TDI released a fiery press release stating that its application "clearly showed otherwise." Despite the loss, insurers in Texas do not appear to have turned to the politics of dissent. Relying on evidence that 92 percent of Texas consumers who purchased policies on the individual market received rebates from MLR reform, some commentators have speculated that any other bona fide challenge to federal policy would be difficult to make.[96]

Diverging Paths to Consent in Connecticut and Indiana

By 2014, both Connecticut and Indiana had come into compliance with the ACA's early market reforms and effective rate review provisions. Yet, illustrating the importance of preexisting policy legacies and low institutional fragmentation, the states took two very different paths to get there. Though many of the early market reforms were popular in both states, and rate review provisions were of particularly low salience, a Democratic governor and state legislature made it much easier for Connecticut to enact new legislation to comply with the reforms.[97] After a debate that pitted unions and health reformers against local chambers of commerce and insurers over whether Connecticut would develop a "public option," in July 2011 Connecticut adopted a broad legislative package enacting the ACA's early market reforms by comfortable legislative margins (eighty-eight to forty-eight in the House; twenty-two to fourteen in the Senate).[98] Prior to the passage of the ACA, Connecticut had passed rate review legislation that satisfied new federal requirements. In July 2011, the state also passed legislation to enhance the Connecticut rate review process beyond the new federal minimum, but Governor Dannel P. Malloy vetoed the bill, reasoning, "The Connecticut Department of Insurance already conducts an objective actuarial analysis of each and every rate increase request."[99] Between 2011 and 2014, Connecticut's insurance commissioner lived up to Malloy's claim. In this period, Connecticut began reviewing and challenging a number of rate increases.[100] In 2014, the Department of Insurance challenge of an average rate increase of 12.75 percent proposed by Anthem Blue Cross Blue Shield led to rate decreases for most consumers on these plans.[101] Therefore, though Connecticut had difficulty expanding beyond the new standards set by the ACA, the partisan makeup of the state and existing decisions made it easier for Connecticut to consent to new federal rules.

In Indiana, the process worked differently. In 2005, its Republican governor, Mitch Daniels, had pushed for legislation eliminating requirements that insurers cover consumers with some preexisting conditions.[102] After the passage of the ACA, however, Daniels had quietly accepted grants from HHS and had planned to establish an insurance exchange but faced pressure from a hostile state legislature and attacks from potential primary challengers on the right. The *National Review* excoriated Daniels for being an "anchor" on the repeal movement.[103] Thus, passing major legislation endorsing the ACA was a nonstarter.

Yet Indiana ultimately consented to the ACA's regulatory reforms *without* having to pass high-profile statutes endorsing the new law, as in the case of the exchanges. Because Indiana already had basic consumer protection and rate review laws on the books, Stephen Robertson, the state insurance commissioner, began using his existing authority to review health insurance products to ensure ACA compliance.[104] Because HHS had not pushed a hard line on the federal minimum standards, the Indiana legislature had to do little else to bring the state into compliance with the reform.

This did not sit well with the ACA's partisan opponents. In April 2011, Republicans in the Indiana House passed a bill that would have prohibited Robertson from taking any action whatsoever to implement the ACA, including instituting regulatory reforms under existing Indiana laws.[105] Whereas the House passed this provision sixty-five to thirty-one, the Senate opposed it, insisting on its own language, which preserved Robertson's authority and built on existing Indiana law to prohibit retroactive cancellations of health insurance policies, extend dependent coverage to those under the age of twenty-six, and ban the denial of coverage to children based on preexisting conditions.[106] What emerged from conference committee deliberations was a bill that symbolically "nullified" the ACA's individual mandate provisions but modestly expanded Robertson's authority.[107] This bill became Public Law 160-2011 after House and Senate conferees approved it in May 2011 (sixty-one to thirty-five in the House; twenty-eight to twenty-one in the Senate).[108]

If the road to consent on early market reforms was rocky at times, the Indiana path to consent on rate review was better paved by its strong preexisting policy legacies and the low institutional fragmentation of these provisions. In June 2011, after rate review rules had been finalized and Indiana had sought approval for its rate review program from HHS, Robertson issued a press release claiming, "For more than two decades, Indiana has exercised its authority to review and approve premiums for health insurance policies sold to Hoosiers. Since then, former Commissioners appointed by governors from both political parties have improved the rate review process here in Indiana to what it is today, which actually exceeds the standards required in President Obama's health care law."[109]

Robertson thus simultaneously scored political points as a critic of "Obamacare" while defending Indiana laws that furthered the goals of health care reform. Unsurprisingly, Indiana met federal minimum standards and, given that no additional legislation was necessary, Robertson conducted reviews of premium increases above 10 percent. In 2012 alone, Indiana conducted reviews of six rate increases over 10 percent, five of which led to modification and one of which led the insurer to withdraw the increase altogether.[110] Although opponents of the ACA in Indiana attempted to stall efforts at cooperation, they faced an uphill battle. As the next section suggests, this was the prevailing pattern in the politics of regulatory reform.

THE POLITICS OF DISSENT

When conservative group ALEC published the *State Legislators Guide to Repealing ObamaCare* in 2011, it strongly attacked what it called the "federal takeover of health insurance legislation." As the guide put it, the ACA's new regulatory reforms "not only restrict states' ability to regulate health plans but they also override patient protections already adopted by the states."[111] With a much more competitive political environment after the 2010 elections, ALEC's advice to opponents of regulatory reform was to refuse federal rate review grants that "conscript states as arms of federal policy."[112] The guide also suggested that state legislators create an "interstate health compact" that would assert the primacy of the states in regulating health insurance markets. Finally, ALEC urged state legislators to author bills to reduce the authority of insurance commissioners to enforce new regulations on the insurance market, including the ban on insurer discrimination against sick patients.[113]

Yet as Figure 5.3 shows, only five states—Alabama, Missouri, Oklahoma, Texas, and Wyoming—effectively dissented from the early market reforms and rate review. Despite ALEC's strong push for state resistance to new regulatory policy, would-be dissenters faced roadblocks. In almost every case, state departments of insurance had the ability to carry out regulatory reforms without further legislative action, preempting opponents from using state-level legislative veto points to contest the ACA. Even when new reforms would have required adjustments by state legislatures, the law's core regulatory provisions directed opponents' attention to intergovernmental bargaining between HHS and state insurance regulators

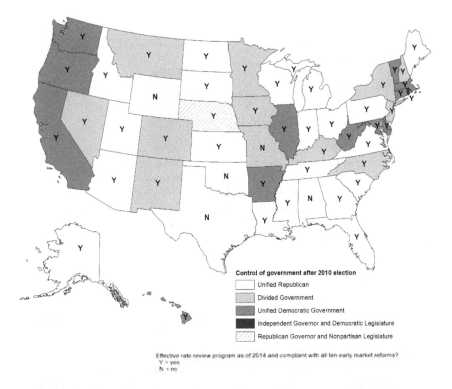

Figure 5.3 State Decisions on Early Market Reforms and Rate Review as of April 2014

Note: Partisan control in Iowa, Kansas, Louisiana, Mississippi, New Jersey, New Mexico, South Carolina, and Virginia reflects 2011 off-cycle or special-election results.

Source: Katie Keith and Kevin Lucia, *Implementing the Affordable Care Act: The State of the States,* Commonwealth Fund Brief (New York: Commonwealth Fund, 2014), 13. Partisan control data compiled by authors from Ballotpedia.com.

rather than to legislatures. Furthermore, the ACA's regulatory provisions were not especially salient to consumers. The few salient ones enjoyed some measure of public support that raised even more barriers to the kinds of symbolic politics we saw with the exchanges and Medicaid expansion. The politics of dissent was thus highly attenuated, as we detail in the next section.

Limited State-Level Challenges to the ACA's Regulatory Reforms

Although strong partisan and ideological motivations may have evoked "tough talk" from opponents of the ACA, it was not always easy to push state governments toward dissent. In the cases of Medicaid expansion and the exchanges, dissent was

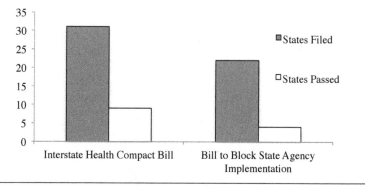

Figure 5.4 Attempts to Block State Cooperation with Regulatory Reforms, 2011–2014
Source: National Conference of State Legislatures, "State Laws and Actions Challenging Certain Health Reforms," accessed October 14, 2014, http://www.ncsl.org/research/health/state-laws-and-actions-challenging-ppaca.aspx.

easier because it required only inaction. With weak policy legacies and fragmented institutions, opponents merely had to use the veto points of the state legislative process to *block* legislation to adopt the exchanges and Medicaid expansion. Yet early on in the rollout of the ACA's regulatory reforms, organizations such as ALEC realized that insurance commissioners could act under their existing authority to start the ball rolling. Insurance commissioners in nearly all states, including the five that eventually refused to comply with the ACA's early market reforms and rate review provisions, initially cooperated with HHS, conducting reviews or issuing subregulatory guidance. Yet to stop this from happening, opponents of the ACA had to take action, which proved difficult.

To stall state agencies from implementing the reforms, legislators in thirty-one states attempted to create an "interstate health insurance compact" that would have asserted the authority of the states alone to regulate the insurance market (see Figure 5.4). Yet only nine states passed compact bills. Even these bills turned out to operate at a symbolic level because congressional approval was still required to make the interstate compact law.[114]

More concretely, legislators in twenty-two states attempted to block state agency implementation of federal regulations. As the previous discussion of the Indiana attempt suggests, however, bills to rescind existing authority often proved unpopular; to date only four states have passed such measures. After the ACA passed, insurance commissioners in three of these states, Missouri, Oklahoma, and Wyoming, reported that they would no longer enforce the ACA's market reforms through subregulatory guidance. Although Alabama and Texas did not pass similar legislation, insurance commissioners in these two states abandoned their initial cooperative approach to implementing market reforms after opposition to the ACA heated up in 2012. By April 2013, Jim Ridling, the Alabama insurance commissioner, issued a bulletin directing insurers to submit their products to CCIIO for review.[115] In August, a spokesperson for the Texas Department of Insurance reported, "We can't act on anything that doesn't exist in state law."[116] For opponents of the ACA's market reforms in most states, however, legislative change was necessary and, as Figure 5.4 suggests, difficult to achieve.

Opponents of MLR and rate review provisions fared no better. Of the thirty-nine state bill introductions related to the MLR between 2011 and 2013, only six involved "challenges" to the reform. None of these bills attempted to symbolically nullify the MLR. A failed 2011 bill introduced in Georgia, for instance, directed the governor to apply for a federal regulatory waiver.[117] Another stillborn bill, this time in New Jersey (a state with a divided government), permitted health maintenance organizations to include charity care assessments for the purposes of meeting certain MLR requirements of 85 percent for large-group policies and 80 percent for small-group plans.[118] Regarding rate review, only three bills were introduced between 2011 and 2013 to challenge the ACA's reforms.[119] Of these, only one made its way through the legislature. Tennessee enacted legislation to weaken rate review provisions, providing that premium estimates released by insurers "shall not require a policy form, rate filing, or approval by the commissioner of commerce and insurance."[120] Yet this legislation did not move Tennessee "out of compliance" with federal rate review policy.[121]

One additional insight into the politics of dissent is how states interacted with federal grants to improve their rate review processes. The ACA established a five-year premium rate review grant program beginning in 2010, appropriating $250 million for HHS to award grants to states from fiscal year 2010 through 2014.[122] Under this authority, HHS created two grant cycles in which states could apply for funds for a variety of purposes, including developing systems for cataloguing and making public rate reviews and filings, developing better information technology for analyzing and cataloguing rate filings, and hiring new actuarial staff.[123]

Rate review grants did not appear innocuous to opponents of the ACA. Accepting federal dollars meant regular oversight of state activities on rate review, including quarterly progress reports, weekly project reports, regular phone communication between federal and state officials, and annual audits.[124] Yet as early as August 2010, forty-five of fifty states had received more than $46 million in grant funds. Among these were a sizable number of states in which opposition to the ACA ran high, including nineteen of the twenty-two states suing HHS over health care reform in the federal courts. Virginia, whose attorney general led the legal charge against health care reform, applied for a $1 million grant to expand the amount of information required for insurance companies to provide when they filed their rates with the state and to develop a new procedural manual for rate fil-ing.[125] By the end of the grant process, only four states (Alaska, Georgia, Iowa, and Wyoming) had not filed any grant applications.

In 2011, ALEC and conservative legislators in the states sought to reverse this trend. In its guide to repealing Obamacare, ALEC suggested that opposing the ACA meant that states should refuse these grants as a matter of political prin-ciple.[126] Though states had already accepted them, ALEC's message persuaded sev-eral legislatures and governors to return rate review funds to HHS. In addition to the four states that refused the funds initially, an additional six returned more than 50 percent of their funds. Notably, Florida returned $1 million in federal grants for rate review enhancement in 2011; Oklahoma returned nearly the same amount that year.[127] States with unified Republican government returned an average of 22 percent of their rate review funds. This was only slightly higher than states with unified Democratic government, which returned an average of 16 percent of rate review grants each. Yet as the evidence in Chapter 3 suggests, differences between states were minor, especially when compared with state returns of grants to plan and establish health insurance exchanges. To better understand the differences that led the small group of five states to engage in dissent, we compare the politics of regulatory reform in Arizona and Missouri.

The Politics of Dissent in Arizona and Missouri

Arizona and Missouri provide a good basis for understanding the challenges of dissent. Opponents of the ACA in both states lobbied against implementation of the ACA's regulatory provisions, and the Missouri General Assembly ultimately passed a law in 2011 that stalled cooperation on either rate review or the early market reforms; in contrast, after some delay, Arizona cooperated on both reforms despite pressure from the state legislature to do otherwise. What made the differ-ence was not only the strength of the opposition but also how opponents of health reform packaged their opposition to overcome state legislative veto points.

In 2010, Missouri may not have looked like the typical state that would re-fuse to participate in the ACA's regulatory reforms. In September, the director of the Missouri Department of Insurance, John Huff, issued a bulletin to insurers informing them of the department's compliance with the ACA's early market re-forms and his intention to begin reviewing health insurance policies to ensure compliance.[128] Governor Jay Nixon, a Democrat, had appointed Huff to his post in 2011. Although Huff still lacked rate review authority in the individual market, Missouri applied for a $1 million rate review grant from the CMS to construct a data system for reviewing premium increases from scratch, develop a consumer-friendly website for posting rate increases, and expand the state capacity and authority to conduct reviews.[129]

Yet cooperation with the ACA was cut short by a Republican-led attack in the Missouri legislature. Representative Denny Hoskins (R-Warrensburg) led the attack. Unlike legislation in other state assemblies, Hoskins's bill was carefully calibrated to navigate the veto points of the state legislative process. Rather than introducing a new piece of legislation, Hoskins styled his bill as a series of amendments to the 2009 "Big Government Get Off My Back Act," designed deliberately to appeal to Democrats, especially the governor, who Republicans had cornered on the issue of job creation. As drafted, Hoskins's bill hitched new constraints on cooperation with the ACA to popular small-business tax deductions from the 2009 bill. Moreover, the new legislation did not *explicitly* erase Missouri authority to cooperate with federal officials in implementing the ACA. Rather, it specified that any implementation of federal mandates that Missouri Republicans pegged as "job killers" would have to be specifically authorized by the legislature.

In practice, these provisions would make it difficult for the Missouri Department of Insurance to act within its already limited existing authority to review insurance policies and rate increases. Yet Hoskins's design was ingenious; the bill moved quickly through the House with a final vote of 136–21. By the time Nixon gave his State of the State address in late January 2011, Hoskins celebrated that the "Governor is in agreement with the General Assembly that it is imperative to put Missourians back to work and maintain a balanced budget."[130] Indeed, the popular tax deductions had made Hoskins's proposal irresistible. After additional deliberation and only minor modifications in the Senate, the bill passed unanimously (thirty-four to zero) in April 2011.[131]

Newspapers covering the passage of Hoskins's bill through the state legislature referred to it only as a "small-business tax break." As Hoskins put it in May 2011, "It's basically a job and economic tool for Main Street, not for Wall Street."[132] By the end of the Missouri legislative session, the bill had received Nixon's signature, and with it, the end of cooperation on the ACA's regulatory reforms. As of 2013, Missouri had returned all but $91,072 of its initial rate review grant.[133] In short order, Huff's department ceased to review insurance products, claiming that it no longer had the authority to do so.[134] Yet stalling cooperation had depended not merely on hostility toward "Obamacare" or the insurance commissioner but the attachment of a proposal to limit state authority on an already popular legislative proposal.

As the case of Arizona shows, challenging the ACA's regulatory reforms was more difficult without cleverly designed legislation. Following the passage of the ACA, Arizona was slow to take action on regulatory reforms. Germaine Marks, the Arizona insurance commissioner, had failed to report any compliance activities by 2012.[135] Yet if Republican governor Jan Brewer was uncertain about consenting to the reform, she was equally uncertain about dissent. When the state legislature passed an interstate compact challenging the ACA's regulatory reforms in 2011, Brewer vetoed it.[136] In her veto message, the governor claimed that the bill violated the separation of powers in the Arizona Constitution and would result in "additional fiscal challenges for our health care system."[137] By 2013, Republicans in the state legislature had failed to muster a majority for a similar bill to challenge the state compliance with the ACA. Instead, with mounting pressure from insurers and public interest organizations alike, the legislature passed—by a comfortable margin—a blanket policy (HB 2550) that directed the insurance commissioner to ensure that the state "retains its ability" to regulate health insurance.[138] Although the law contained no specific compliance measures, its passage gave Marks the discretion she needed to begin regulating health insurance policies.[139]

Marks had been slow to develop an effective rate review program. After the passage of the ACA and through the end of 2012, federal officials at CCIIO conducted reviews of rate increases for insurers operating in Arizona.[140] Yet this was not because Marks lacked the authority to alter the Arizona rate review process. Throughout 2011 and 2012, she used rate review grants from the CMS to create programs to train staff to use the System for Electronic Rate and Form Filing (SERFF), improve consumer access to rate filings, and hire actuarial consulting firms to evaluate Arizona processes.[141] Conferences held by Marks's department allowed industry stakeholders and consumers to discuss new forms and gather comments for revision.[142] As part of the terms of the Arizona rate review grant, Marks sent confirmation of these activities to CCIIO, which determined that the Arizona program was "effective" in December 2012.[143] She did not need any additional legislative authority from Arizona to establish the program. Instead, Marks issued a bulletin explaining that her department would begin to review premium increases above 10 percent pursuant to an existing chapter of the Arizona Administrative Code.[144] The prior policy history of Arizona, combined with the flexible design of the ACA's provisions, stacked the deck against opponents wishing to challenge the participation of Arizona in the rate review program.

Subterranean Dissent?

If dissent refers to high-visibility decisions at the state level to announce a stance against a federal law, the ACA's regulatory reforms do not seem exemplary. Yet this does not take into account the kinds of nonenforcement actions ALEC described in its guide to state legislators, including state regulatory agencies' failure to exercise their authority to conduct "effective rate review" and to review insurers' conduct to ensure compliance with the ACA's market reforms. Although there is

Table 5.3 Rate Review Outcomes, 2013

	Small-Group Market		Individual Market	
	Requested	Implemented	Requested	Implemented
Number of rate filings	1,099	1,099	647	647
Filings with change rate requested ≥10%	20.7%	18.1%	25%	23.1%
Average rate change	8.0%	7.1%	11.2%	10.3%

Source: US Department of Health and Human Services, *Rate Review Annual Report* (Washington, DC: Government Printing Office, 2014), 5, 7.

evidence of this kind of regulatory "drift,"[145] a pattern in the ACA that warrants further research, there is not enough evidence to discount our argument that regulatory reform invited a quieter politics of negotiated consent.[146]

One potential site of drift may be insurance commissioners' failure to effectively compel insurers to modify their rates in states where partisan and interest group opponents of the ACA were well mobilized. In particular, we might have expected nonenforcement in states that opposed the ACA's other reforms but met the minimum federal requirements for effective rate review programs. Yet as early as 2011, a Kaiser Family Foundation analysis of state rate reviews revealed that state insurance departments—including states where opposition to other parts of the ACA runs high—determined that the vast majority of rate increases in excess of 10 percent were ruled unreasonable. This was true for all requests for rate increases in excess of 10 percent, such as in Alabama, Louisiana, Nebraska, Virginia, and Wisconsin.[147]

State insurance commissioners also appeared to be effectively using their authority. As a 2014 report suggests, insurers in states receiving federal rate review grants requested premium rate increases above the 10 percent threshold infrequently—20 percent of the time in the small-group market and 25 percent of the time in the individual market (see Table 5.3). The average requested rate changes in both markets were also low. Most importantly, however, average implemented rates were lower than requested rates across both markets, indicating that insurance commissioners were making effective use of their authority. This marks a decisive shift from the pre-ACA period. As a recent study from the University of Chicago shows, premium increases in a sample of states slowed substantially after the ACA rate regulations took hold. In the individual market, premium increases fell from 11.7 percent in 2010 to 7.1 percent in 2012. In the small-group market, increases diminished from 8.8 percent in 2010 to 4.8 percent in 2012.[148] Although rate review processes may require improvement in some states, initial evidence suggests rate review is not a site of "subterranean dissent."

Another potential opportunity for drift is the failure of state departments of insurance to adequately review and approve insurance products available in new health insurance exchanges. Yet with the exception of the five states that have refused to comply with early market reforms, there is little evidence state regulators have been deliberately stalling the review and approval of plans. A recent study by researchers at Georgetown University revealed, for instance, that even states without their own insurance exchanges have "adapted to new requirements to review plans for discriminatory benefit designs and coverage of habilitative services."[149]

Another likely scenario for regulatory drift is the failure of state insurance departments to assist the uninsured in learning about coverage options and guaranteed benefits. In 2014, an Urban Institute study revealed that the majority of consumers, especially low-income consumers, had heard "nothing at all" about core provisions of the ACA, including the availability of preventive care without copayments or coinsurance and the elimination of dollar limits on coverage for essential health benefits.[150] Because lack of awareness about policy benefits among potential beneficiaries contributes to weaker support, it stands to reason that opponents of the ACA would simply hold back their efforts to provide consumers information about the law. Under the ACA, states have the opportunity to receive federal grants to establish consumer assistance programs (CAPs) designed to help consumers file complaints and appeals about coverage and enroll in qualified health plans and to track problems in access to high-quality coverage.[151] Although the law provided $30 million in grants to the states to take on this function initially and "such sums as may be necessary" in subsequent years, a cash-strapped HHS has found it difficult to keep the program going.

In a constrained fiscal context, most states that initially operated a CAP have discontinued it, as Table 5.4 shows. In many states where opposition to the ACA ran high, governors such as Pat McCrory of North Carolina refused to provide state money to continue the program.[152] Yet potential drift in CAPs is not particular to states where opposition to the ACA is strong. As of 2014, only fifteen states continued to operate CAPs, suggesting a potential challenge for raising consumer awareness about the ACA's market reforms and generating effective consumer complaints about insurer practices that violate health care reform. Although the ACA provides additional funding for nonprofit organizations to become health insurance "navigators," these organizations have been overburdened with addressing eligibility determination decisions and continue to depend on state governments for assistance.[153] It is too soon to tell what the future holds for state efforts at consumer outreach, yet this is one potential area in which opponents of the ACA could leverage opportunities for subterranean dissent.

Table 5.4 Consumer Assistance Programs in the States, 2014

Never applied for federal funds	AK, AL, AZ, CO, HI, ID, IN, KS, LA, ND, NE, NV, OH, SD, TN, UT, WI, WY
Program discontinued	AR, DE, FL, GA, IA, MT, NH, NJ, OK, OR, PA, RI, SC, TX, VA, WA, WV
In operation	CA, CT, IL,* KY,* MA, MD, ME, MI, MN, MO, MS, NC, NM, NY, VT

*State operates its own program without federal assistance.

Source: Centers for Medicare and Medicaid Services, Consumer Assistance Programs, accessed October 24, 2014, http://www.cms.gov/CCIIO/Resources/Consumer-Assistance-Grants/.

The potential for drift aside, our evidence suggests opponents of the ACA faced real limits to dissent on regulatory reform. Opponents had to take positive action to circumscribe the authority of state regulators, which foreclosed effective dissent in the legislative process. Finally, although the potential for regulatory drift exists, evidence of subterranean dissent is modest at best.

CONCLUSION

The ACA's regulatory reforms are by no means faits accomplis—that is, immune to future political battles. Federal regulations could ostensibly be overturned by a future presidential administration, and state cooperation, given the right conditions, could turn into dissent. Yet the evidence presented here suggests the regulatory politics of the ACA proceeded along a trajectory that differs from the ones we have described in the past two chapters. First, opponents of the ACA faced limits in pursuing the politics of dissent. Despite its opposition to some details of the reforms, the insurance industry has generally worked through the intergovernmental bargaining process rather than pushing for legislative obstruction at the state level. Moreover, partisan and ideological opponents have also found it difficult to entirely obstruct the ACA's reforms in all but a handful of states. Preexisting legacies of state engagement on insurance regulation, combined with statutory provisions that did not generally require positive action by state legislatures, channeled debates over regulation into bureaucratic venues, which meant that opponents did not generally have access to high-profile political venues where dissent is usually lodged. The complexity of regulatory reforms does not appear to have helped in this regard. Low salience combined with strong public support for these reforms did not allow for the kind of symbolic politics on which dissent hinges.

Second, the absence of high-profile legislative battles at the state level has not meant the absence of opponents' political engagement. Rather, the structure of the ACA's regulatory reforms and the preexisting legacy of state authority over insurance regulation gave opponents opportunities to engage in intergovernmental bargaining. One consequence of opponents' early mobilization against the ACA is that state and federal regulators were under pressure to "lower the floor" on early market reforms and rate review provisions such that states did not have to enshrine the goals of the ACA in their statute books. With MLR reform, however, opponents of the ACA did not enjoy such influence on the process, and little "floor lowering" occurred.

In explaining the difference between MLR and rate review, it is hard to overstate the role of the congressional MLR defenders who pressured the NAIC and HHS alike to honor their specific intentions in developing strong, uniform national standards. The attentiveness of Senator Rockefeller to intergovernmental bargaining ultimately brought many state regulators to support stronger national standards. Though the insurance industry can be seen as an institutional loser in the debate over final MLR rules, it has continued to mobilize at the state level, using the waiver process to do so. Although states such as Texas have been unsuccessful in pursuing federal waivers and seem unlikely to challenge MLR provisions as long as consumers continue to receive rebates, changes in the partisan composition of the executive branch and Congress could still reverse these policy gains. Despite whatever partisan turnovers occur, it would appear that the future of ACA's major regulatory reforms lies in a quieter politics of bargaining and consent, in sharp contrast to the politics of dissent so dominant in state implementation of exchanges and Medicaid expansion.

Conclusion

The Patient Protection and Affordable Care Act (ACA) is the most important health care reform in the United States in more than forty years, and it is likely to remain a subject of political controversy in the near future. Yet the political environment of health care reform implementation is not monolithic. Rather, the ACA is a complex bundle of distinct reform streams, each characterized by a distinctive political and institutional logic. As our analyses of health insurance exchanges, Medicaid expansion, and regulatory reform suggest, the political battles over implementing health care reform are as diverse as the policy issues embedded in the legislation itself. It would be insufficient, our evidence shows, to suggest that partisan polarization alone has driven state government responses to the ACA. Rather, by shifting the unit of analysis from states to reform streams, we show how three factors—policy legacies, level of institutional fragmentation, and public sentiments—explain political differences among these key components of the ACA. In this short conclusion, we return to our framework, reflecting on how it helps us to explain the ACA's postreform politics before exploring the broad analytical contributions of our study.

WHAT EXPLAINS DIVERGENCE AMONG THE CASES?

By tracking the role of the states in implementing health care policy, our analysis compared and contrasted the politics of federalism in three distinct reform streams: health insurance exchanges, Medicaid expansion, and regulatory reform. The first striking aspect of our analysis is the variety of political maneuvers used in the different streams during implementation. As demonstrated, health insurance exchanges and Medicaid expansion exhibit much greater political conflict in the states than regulatory reform. Importantly, each reform stream involves different actors and diverse forms of policy bargaining and political dissent. To explain the differences between our three cases, our analysis focuses on three main factors: policy legacies, institutional fragmentation, and public sentiments.

First, policy legacies are crucial in explaining varying postenactment politics in each of the three reform streams. Our analysis suggests that, in terms of policy legacies, one especially significant factor is whether robust preexisting state or federal policies create a basis on which state governments can negotiate their consent. This analysis points to the fact that health insurance exchanges were the least-developed institutions of the three streams because of their relatively recent creation, especially compared with Medicaid, a program that since its inception in 1965 has established well-structured policy legacies and intergovernmental channels. Without preexisting authority, states that wished to create health insurance exchanges had to take positive legislative action, a move that proved controversial especially in the Republican-dominated policy environment in the states. In the case of Medicaid expansion, a legacy of "executive federalism"—bargaining between federal and state officials—permitted some governors to negotiate alternatives to expanding the traditional Medicaid program, a trend that may continue to develop gradually over time. Although less developed than Medicaid in terms of a federal-state relationship, the regulatory reform stream is characterized by more established state policy legacies than the health insurance exchange stream, which greatly facilitates the negotiation of consent central to regulatory reform in the context of ACA implementation and intergovernmental relations. With well-developed policy networks and existing statutory authority to regulate the insurance market, state regulators can bargain over the federal policy "floor" such that new federal regulations accommodate the diversity of existing state approaches to reform, minimizing dissenting actions.

Second, levels of institutional fragmentation vary significantly across our three reform streams, a phenomenon that directly affects the intergovernmental politics of implementation. Regulatory reform is the least fragmented of the three streams under consideration because the ACA's regulatory reforms did not require most state legislatures to create new authority. In reforms such as the ACA's rate review provision, states implement minimum federal standards or face the prospect of preemption by the Department of Health and Human Services (HHS); in the case of the medical loss ratio (MLR), states have no direct implementation role. This means state and federal regulators can negotiate policy under the political radar without raising the specter of contentious state legislative debates. On the other end of the fragmentation spectrum are health insurance exchanges, which constitute a balkanized policy environment with weaker fiscal incentives and few preexisting frameworks on which to build. This situation provides states more institutional leverage to reject participation (in this case, in the creation of their own exchanges). In contrast, within the Medicaid expansion stream, states have a direct fiscal incentive to participate in reforming the program, but as a result of the 2012 Supreme Court decision in *National Federation of Independent Business (NFIB) v. Sebelius* are not compelled to do so.

Finally, the contrasts among our three reform streams are just as strong when we turn to public sentiments. As our analysis shows, the clear outlier here is once again regulatory reform, a low-profile policy stream that typically remains insulated from extensive, high-profile media coverage, a situation that provides much less room for public controversy and symbolic politics. In the context of divided public sentiments toward the ACA as a whole, it becomes clear from our analysis that both Medicaid expansion and the health insurance exchanges are much more visible issues. State politicians and advocates frame these issues within their own ideological views about health care reform and often make them visible to citizens and the various constituencies they represent by using symbolic politics. Clearly, in the case of health insurance exchanges and Medicaid expansion (and in contrast to regulatory reform), high visibility combined with divided public sentiments and the capacity of opponents to use symbolic politics to stir discontent about the ACA exacerbate political conflict in state and intergovernmental policy making over the implementation of health insurance reform.

Taken together, these three factors explain why health insurance exchanges—the reform stream with the weakest policy legacies, the most fragmented policy environment, limited financial incentives for the states, and a high level of public consciousness—feature the highest degree of state-level dissent. Indeed, most states, including the vast majority of Republican-controlled states, have refused to create their own health insurance exchanges, creating a major—and initially unanticipated—fiscal and political burden for the federal government. As for Medicaid expansion, this policy stream features better-rooted policy legacies, a less-fragmented institutional setting, and clear fiscal incentives that motivate states to comply, which helps account for the fact that more states agreed to expand Medicaid than to set up their own exchanges. Medicaid, however, is a highly visible and politically divisive program that cannot be expanded without executive and in most cases legislative action. This is a key difference between both Medicaid expansion and health insurance exchanges and regulatory reform, a stream where bargaining behind closed doors among federal and state officials is the norm, a situation that helps reduce the level of public dissent over this aspect of the ACA.

Our three factors provide a richer explanation for state government engagement in the politics of consent or dissent in the case of the ACA than the reigning conventional wisdom about the ACA, which focuses on the single factor of partisan polarization. This is not because partisan control of state government or the policy preferences of state officials do not matter. Indeed, one has only to look at the implementation maps featured in this book to comprehend the dramatic extent to which partisan control separates states that chose to cooperate from those that did not. Yet partisanship and polarization perform poorly in explaining why all but four states with unified Republican government ultimately complied with the ACA's regulatory reforms and why an increasing number of such states appear to be moving toward some form of Medicaid expansion. Indeed, we can account for these deviations from the partisan pattern we observe in the case of exchanges by referencing the historical, institutional, and public opinion contexts we have laid out here. The ACA is not a coherent, unified reform but rather a set of reform streams, each characterized by a distinct type of politics.

Although we have provided considerable evidence supporting our claims, scholars may disagree with our interpretation, offering their own explanations of the political differences we have observed among our three reform streams. For instance, some may reason that exchanges foster less cooperation than our two other reform streams simply because they are seen as being closely linked to the individual mandate, a controversial aspect of the ACA onto which opponents more quickly latched. This reasoning, however, ignores the fact that health insurance exchanges did not prove controversial at all during the enactment process, as we suggested in Chapter 3. In this context, the controversy around exchanges is not a spontaneous reaction to the nature of certain policy provisions. Even more, proponents may argue that regulatory reform is less controversial than both Medicaid expansion and the creation of exchanges because opponents care less about this issue. There is certainly interest in regulatory reform among stakeholders, including opponents of the ACA, as we addressed in Chapter 2. Yet, in this reform stream, because of the three factors we highlight, it makes more sense for policy actors to seek negotiated consent behind closed doors rather than staging a public campaign against the reforms.

THEORETICAL IMPLICATIONS

Our analysis has profound implications for how we understand the link between federalism and the politics of public policy. First, this book contributes to the literature on postreform politics, which suggests that a reform can significantly change even *after* it has been enacted. As Eric Patashnik argues, politics endures even beyond the bill's initiation into law.[1] However, this idea of postreform politics lacks attention to the nuances of federalism and state politics.[2] Whereas other scholars have shown the ways in which market reforms invite backlash in their failure to sufficiently restructure the interest-group landscape, we argue that reforms can actually create room for opponents to exercise their dissent because federalism often diffuses power when requiring ratification of initiatives by governors and state legislatures. Especially under conditions of intense policy conflict, these actors hold veto powers that facilitate the diffusion of national policy. It is true, however, that federalism does not *always* give opponents enough leverage to challenge reforms. As Frank Thompson's work on Medicaid has shown, the involvement of state governments in the program over time has created the capacity for innovation and institutional resilience.[3] Still, very little literature exists explaining the conditions in which the fragmentation of power stabilizes and destabilizes new reforms.

Second, this book makes a direct contribution to the literature on what scholars call the "varieties of federalism," which refers mainly to the fact that federal systems vary greatly from one country to the next. For instance, even federal countries
that may appear to have a good deal in common, such as Australia, Canada, and
the United States, work quite differently as federal systems.[4] Our analysis, however,
emphasizes the internal variations of federalism that can appear within the same
country and, in our case, even in the same policy domain.[5] Whereas other scholars
have asserted that the politics of federalism can vary across policy sectors—education and environmental policy, for instance—we show that even when focusing
on a single policy change, one can observe highly divergent patterns of politics.[6]
As our comparative analysis suggests, each reform stream under consideration is
characterized by its own distinct form of state politics and intergovernmental relations. To talk about the "politics of federalism" in general is potentially misleading;
politics can change drastically from one aspect of a reform to the next.

Finally, and relatedly, our analysis further contributes to the study of federalism and public policy not only by showing how the politics of federalism varies from one reform stream to another within the same policy area but also by
offering an integrated framework that helps explain why these variations occur
at all. To date, no such integrated framework exists. Although our approach may
require modification when applied to other types of reform, we believe the process
of looking at interactions between policy legacies, levels of institutional fragmentation, and public sentiments sheds meaningful light on the political "varieties of
federalism" within the same policy areas or, at least, within the same country across
different policy areas.

THE LEGACIES OF THE ACA

Because the ACA is a set of heterogeneous policy changes, any discussion about
the future of this legislation should at least in part emphasize trends specific to
each reform stream. This is why, in this last section, we focus primarily on trends
that should prove consequential in the continuing implementation of the ACA.
Our goal here is not to speculate on the long-term political effects of the reform
but simply to draw attention to a few issues that may spark political controversy
in the years ahead.

First, health insurance exchanges are particularly vulnerable to political attacks from within the federal government and may remain a political nonstarter in
Republican-dominated states. Thus, what may be threatening to supporters of the
ACA within the federal government itself could be the prospect of budget battles
resulting in defunding federally operated exchanges. This potential threat is espe-

cially acute because the ACA does not feature adequate fiscal provisions financing the development of such federal exchanges in states. Similar budgetary concerns might also emerge in states that have implemented their own exchanges but where, possibly in the context of state-level electoral shifts, opponents could still try to defund such exchanges.

After a period of considerable tension, however, direct legal challenges to the operation of federal exchanges in Republican states may have subsided. In July 2014, a federal appeals court ruled that "said language in the Affordable Care Act allows only state-run exchanges to give consumers tax credits to help pay for policy premiums."[7] Yet, eleven months later, in *King v. Burwell*, the Supreme Court refused to uphold that ruling by a vote of six to three. Rather, the Court's majority—led by Chief Justice John Roberts—ruled that tax credits can be paid to consumers via federally run exchanges. This decision prevented potential upheaval for millions of Americans already participating in federal exchanges.[8]

By upholding the federal exchanges in *King*, the Court may have created a more favorable environment for the negotiation of consent in Republican states, where governors or state legislators may have an incentive to create distinct alternatives to the federal marketplace. In particular, states may opt to use innovation waivers under section 1332 of the ACA to experiment with alternative approaches to offering insurance coverage.[9] Importantly, innovation waivers may allow states to introduce alternatives to the individual mandate, such as multiyear waiting periods for those who miss an enrollment deadline and increasing penalties for late enrollment. States could also introduce alternatives to the employer mandate, such as requiring employers to "pay a flat percentage of payroll in benefits or taxes."[10]

Second, the fiscal incentives of Medicaid expansion may create the possibility of gradual adoption over time in the states. Here, money promised by the federal government works as a major incentive for states (even those with unified Republican governments) to cooperate with ACA requirements. As described in Chapter 4, the prospect of federal dollars paved the way for some conflict between Republican governors anxious to take the federal money and Republican state legislators more focused on ideological and partisan imperatives. In the long term, if states persist in nonparticipation in the Medicaid expansion, they will forfeit significant potential revenues. For example, in Florida—where Governor Rick Scott briefly flirted with the idea of expansion until he was knocked back by the legislature—it is estimated that the state would lose $66.1 billion over ten years. Democrats, advocates for low-income Floridians, and the majority of members of the medical industry will pressure the governor to reverse the state position on expansion because only a third of the bill will actually be paid to reimburse hospitals for the care they provide.[11] Similar fiscal logic in other states that had not expanded their

Medicaid programs by 2014 could result, over time, in more states trying to find ways of accommodating to the ACA.

Finally, within regulatory reform, contemporary trends vary significantly from one policy issue to the next. On the one hand, MLR reform has already been relatively successful in helping to keep premiums down, reducing them by about $9 billion between 2011 and 2014.[12] Faced with potentially paying out massive rebates, insurance companies in both individual and small-group markets have improved their compliance with the MLR in the past two years. In 2014, total rebates in the individual market fell to $128 million, down from $192 million in 2013. In the small-group market, rebates fell to $122 million, down from $203 million the previous year.[13] Nevertheless, insurance providers continue to claim that the MLR has not placed downward pressure on premiums and may even increase premiums over time.[14] If insurers prove correct, it may give opponents further ammunition to push for repeal, which the speedy MLR implementation precluded.

The future of other market reforms, however, is more uncertain. To date, five Republican-dominated states have not yet established rate review programs or ACA-compliant market reforms.[15] Even in states such as California where effective rate review programs exist, state insurance regulators do not yet have the authority to reject double-digit rate increases. In November 2014, a state ballot initiative to increase the authority of California to review increases failed by a wide margin.[16] As rate reforms place costs directly on insurance companies and not on consumers, consumer discontent could gradually push insurance companies to keep rates down even if no new reforms are enacted. Yet to the extent that variation remains across states in terms of regulatory regimes, state regulators will have to walk a tightrope, keeping rate increases low to please consumers without risking the exit of insurance companies from their marketplaces.[17] This incremental, state-specific pattern of reform suggests that the politics of rate review will operate primarily in state-level bargains between consumer representatives and insurance companies.

Beyond these policy-specific trends, it is also clear that changing public sentiments around the ACA, on top of partisan shifts at both the state and the federal levels, are likely to affect the future of the law's implementation. At the state level, the 2014 midterm elections have deepened the trend that started in 2010. Republicans gained control of legislative chambers in nine states and flipped Democratic governor's seats in three blue states, including Illinois and Massachusetts.[18] Voters in dark-blue Maryland elected a Republican governor, Larry Hogan, who had made the flawed state insurance exchange a central issue of his campaign.[19] In Arizona, which expanded Medicaid and established effective regulatory reforms, a successful 2014 ballot initiative—Proposition 122—allows (but does not require) the state to restrict the use of personnel to enforce the ACA.[20] The tense environment at the state level is especially likely to affect the health insurance exchanges and Medicaid, currently much less insulated from political battles than regulatory reform.

Second, the results of the 2016 elections could directly affect the fate of the ACA. This is especially true if a Republican enters the White House in the context of GOP majorities in both chambers of Congress. Still, because the ACA has already generated its own vested interests and embedded policy legacies, pure and simple repeal is unlikely. This does not necessarily mean that partisan shifts in Washington may prove inconsequential, in part because of the fiscal and budgetary challenges we have discussed. New challenges in ACA implementation could appear in light of partisan shifts in the states and similar budgetary issues, which would enable Republicans to gain power in previously Democratic states.

Third, proponents of the ACA both within and outside of the Obama administration have long claimed that public support for the legislation would gradually improve as the concrete benefits of the law's provisions trickle down and become more apparent to ordinary citizens. So far, this has not been the case because support for the ACA has remained mixed, a situation related to strong partisan divide over the issue. According to the Kaiser Family Foundation, in late May 2014, 62 percent of Democrats held a positive view of the ACA compared with a mere 12 percent of Republicans. These enduring negative public sentiments among Republican supporters help explain why, in late May 2014, only 37 percent of Americans viewed the law positively, compared with 53 percent who had a negative view of it.[21] Although a number of major ACA provisions were implemented by the time this public opinion data was gathered, one could argue that more time is necessary for citizens to experience and assess the potential benefits of these provisions. However, the close relationship between partisan leanings and perceptions of the ACA may suggest that divided public sentiments about the legislation are likely to endure.

Although we cannot make predictions about the law's political future, our analysis serves an important purpose by explaining the ACA's present. Our account should inform the ongoing public debate over health care reform by identifying the key stakeholders, decisions, and institutional venues in which politics will continue to play out—as well as the historical processes that have shaped current debates. Further, we hope our analysis of the interaction among policy legacies, institutional settings, and public sentiments helps scholars to grasp the political logics surrounding health care reform as well as the challenges of policy implementation in a fragmented federal system. The ACA is a complex, living laboratory for the analysis of federalism and the politics of implementation. In the years to come as the law evolves, we hope our book remains a useful resource for scholars and policy makers seeking to study heath reform.

NOTES

1. Rosalind S. Helderman, "Cuccinelli Sues Federal Government to Stop Health-Care Reform Law," *Washington Post*, March 24, 2010, http://www.washingtonpost.com/wp-dyn/content/article /2010/03/23/AR2010032304224.html.

2. Linda Greenhouse, "By Any Means Necessary," *New York Times*, August 20, 2014, accessed October 23, 2014, http://www.nytimes.com/2014/08/21/opinion/linda-greenhouse-by-any-means -necessary.html?smid=fb-share&_r=0. Greve's statement can be viewed here: "Who's in Charge? More Legal Challenges to the Patient Protection and Affordable Care Act," American Enterprise Institute, last modified December 6, 2010, accessed October 24, 2014, http://aei.org/article/health /healthcare-reform/whos-in-charge-more-legal-challenges-to-the-patient-protection-and -affordable-care-act-event/.

3. Barack Obama, "Remarks by the President on the Affordable Care Act," April 1, 2014, accessed October 24, 2014, http://www.whitehouse.gov/the-press-office/2014/04/01/remarks -president-affordable-care-act.

4. Eric M. Patashnik, *Reforms at Risk: What Happens after Major Policy Changes Are Enacted* (Princeton, NJ: Princeton University Press, 2008).

5. Lawrence R. Jacobs and Theda Skocpol, *Health Care Reform and American Politics: What Everyone Needs to Know* (New York: Oxford University Press, 2010).

6. Eric M. Patashnik and Julian E. Zelizer, "The Struggle to Remake Politics: Liberal Reform and the Limits of Policy Feedback in the Contemporary American State," *Perspectives on Politics* 11, no. 4 (2013): 1071–1087.

7. Ibid.; Kimberly Morgan and Andrea Campbell, "Delegated Governance and the Affordable Care Act," *Journal of Health Policy, Politics, and Law* 36 (June 2011): 387–391; Alan Weil and Raymond Scheppach, "New Roles for States in Health Reform Implementation," *Health Affairs* 26 (June 2010): 1178–1182.

8. The concept of public sentiments is borrowed from John L Campbell, *Institutional Change and Globalization* (Princeton, NJ: Princeton University Press, 2004). Please note that the way we use the term "stream" has nothing to do with the multiple-stream framework in agenda-setting research associated with the work of John W. Kingdon, author of *Agendas, Alternatives, and Public Policies* (Boston: Little, Brown, 1984).

9. William J. Clinton and Al Gore, *Putting People First: A Strategy for Change* (New York: Times Books, 1992), 107.

10. US Bureau of the Census, Statistical Abstract of the United States: 1996, 116th ed. (Washington, DC: Government Printing Office, 1996), 120.

11. Kent Patel and Mark Rushefsky, *Health Care Politics and Policy in America* (Armonk, NY: M. E. Sharpe, 1999), 162.

12. Sven Steinmo and Jon Watts, "It's the Institutions, Stupid! Why Comprehensive National Health Insurance Always Fails in America," *Journal of Health Politics, Policy, and Law* 20, no. 2 (1995): 329–372.

13. Brian K. Atchinson and Daniel M. Fox, "The Politics of the Health Insurance Portability and Accountability Act," *Health Affairs* 16, no. 3 (1997): 146–150.

14. Douglas Jaenicke and Alex Waddan, "President Bush and Social Policy: The Strange Case of the Medicare Prescription Drug Benefit," *Political Science Quarterly* 121, no. 2 (2006): 217–240.

15. L. Brown and M. Sparer, "Poor Program's Progress: The Unanticipated Politics of Medicaid Policy," *Health Affairs* 22, no. 1 (2003): 36.

16. Urban Institute, "State Children's Health Insurance Program," accessed August 31, 2014, http://urban.org/health_policy/medicaid/medicaid-and-schip.cfm.

17. Quoted in Haynes Johnson and David S. Broder, *The System: The American Way of Politics at the Breaking Point* (Boston: Little, Brown, 1996), 651.

18. US Bureau of the Census, "Health Insurance Historical Tables, Table HIB-4: Health Insurance Coverage Status and Type of Coverage by State All People: 1999 to 2012," accessed October 24, 2014, http://www.census.gov/hhes/www/hlthins/data/historical/HIB_tables.html.

19. Deborah Thorne and Elizabeth Warren, "Get Sick, Go Broke," in *Health at Risk: America's Ailing Health System and How to Heal It,* ed. Jacob Hacker (New York: Columbia University Press, 2008), 66–87.

20. Directorate for Employment, Labour, and Social Affairs, "OECD Health Data for 2013," accessed August 31, 2014, http://stats.oecd.org/Index.aspx?DataSetCode=SHA.

21. Congressional Budget Office, *The Budget and Economic Outlook: Fiscal Years 2010 to 2020,* accessed October 24, 2014, http://www.cbo.gov/ftpdocs/108xx/doc10871/01-26-Outlook.pdf.

22. Peter Orszag, "How Health Care Can Save or Sink America," *Foreign Affairs* 90, no. 4 (2011): 42–56. See also Amy Goldstein and Dan Balz, "Governors Differ on Extent of Flexibility for Medicaid," *Washington Post,* February 27, 2011, accessed October 24, 2014, http://www.washington post.com/wp-dyn/content/article/2011/02/27/AR2011022703688.html?wpisrc=nl_politics.

23. The balance between the share of insurance coverage costs paid by employer and employee remained relatively stable through the 2000s. In 1999–2000 at firms offering insurance coverage, employees getting single insurance coverage paid 17.5 percent of costs. By 2010–2011 this had risen to 20.8 percent of premiums. For both employer and employee, however, the cost in dollar terms had gone up significantly because premiums for single coverage "more than doubled." State Health Access Data Assistance Center, *State-Level Trends in Employer-Sponsored Health Insurance* (Minneapolis: University of Minnesota Press, 2013): 11.

24. Charles Morris, *Apart at the Seams: The Collapse of Private Pension and Health Care Protection* (New York: Century Foundation Press, 2006).

25. Marie Gottschalk, "Back to the Future? Health Benefits, Organized Labor, and Universal Health Care," *Journal of Health Policy, Politics, and Law* 32 (2007): 923–970.

26. US Bureau of the Census, "Health Insurance Historical Tables, Table HIB-1: Health Insurance Coverage Status and Type of Coverage by Sex, Race, and Hispanic Origin: 1999 to 2011."

27. Mark Peterson, "It Was a Different Time: Obama and the Unique Opportunity for Health Care Reform," *Journal of Health Politics, Policy, and Law* 36, no. 3 (2011): 429–436.

28. Institute of Medicine, "Unequal Treatment: Confronting Racial and Ethnic Disparities in Health Care," accessed October 24, 2014, http://www.iom.edu/Reports/2002/Unequal-Treatment -Confronting-Racial-and-Ethnic-Disparities-in-Health-Care.aspx.

29. US Bureau of the Census, "Income, Poverty, and Health Insurance Coverage in the United States: 2008" (Washington DC: US Department of Commerce), 21.

30. US Bureau of the Census, "Health Insurance Historical Tables, Table HIB-1."

31. Michael Tesler, "The Spillover of Racialization into Health Care: How President Obama Polarized Public Opinion by Racial Attitudes and Race," *American Journal of Political Science* 56,

no. 3 (2012): 691. Michael Tesler argues that President Obama's race was an important factor in determining attitudes toward health reform. African Americans had long been more supportive than Caucasian Americans of activist government programs, but the differences in attitudes toward policy initiatives increased when Obama entered the White House. Tesler suggests that his findings illustrate that "racial attitudes were both an important determinant of white Americans' health care opinions in the fall of 2009 and that their influence increased significantly *after* President Obama became the face of the policy."

32. Commonwealth Fund, "An Analysis of Survey Data from 11 Countries Finds That 'Satisfaction' with Health System Performance Means Many Things" (2013), accessed March 8, 2015, http://www.commonwealthfund.org/publications/in-brief/2013/apr/survey-data-from-11-countries-finds-that-satisfaction.

33. David K. Jones, Katherine W. V. Bradley, and Jonathan Oberlander, "Pascal's Wager: Health-Insurance Exchanges, Obamacare, and the Republican Dilemma," *Journal of Health Politics, Policy, and Law* 39, no. 1 (2014): 97–137.

34. On the expansion of Medicaid before the advent of the ACA, see Laura K. Olson, *The Politics of Medicaid* (New York: Columbia University Press, 2010).

35. Center for Consumer Information and Insurance Oversight, "Medical Loss Ratio," accessed October 24, 2014, http://www.cms.gov/CCIIO/Programs-and-Initiatives/Health-Insurance-Market-Reforms/Medical-Loss-Ratio.html.

36. See Jones, Bradley, and Oberlander, "Pascal's Wager."

37. Christine Eibner and Evan Saltzman, *The Effect of Eliminating the Affordable Care Act's Tax Credits in Federally Facilitated Marketplaces* (Santa Monica, CA: Rand Corporation, 2015), 5.

38. Ariane de Vogue and Jeremy Diamond, "Supreme Court Saves Obamacare," CNN, June 25, 2015, accessed July 1, 2015, http://www.cnn.com/2015/06/25/politics/supreme-court-ruling-obamacare/.

39. Rachel Garfield, Anthony Damico, Jessica Stephens, and Sahman Rouhani, "The Coverage Gap: Uninsured Poor Adults in States That Do Not Expand Medicaid—an Update," accessed January 10, 2015, http://kff.org/health-reform/issue-brief/the-coverage-gap-uninsured-poor-adults-in-states-that-do-not-expand-medicaid-an-update/.

40. Families U.S.A. "A 50 State Look at Medicaid Expansion," January 28, 2015, accessed March 22, 2015, http://familiesusa.org/product/50-state-look-medicaid-expansion.

41. Katie Keith and Kevin Lucia, *Implementing the Affordable Care Act: The State of the States,* Commonwealth Fund Brief (New York: Commonwealth Fund, 2014).

I. POSTREFORM POLITICS IN THE US FEDERAL SYSTEM

1. America Next, *The Freedom and Empowerment Plan: The Prescription for Conservative Consumer-Focused Health Reform* (Alexandria, VA: America Next, 2014).

2. Jason Millman, "Jindal's Health Plan Starts with a Tough Premise: Repeal All of Obamacare," *Washington Post Wonkblog,* April 2, 2014, accessed April 27, 2014, http://www.washingtonpost.com/blogs/wonkblog/wp/2014/04/02/jindals-health-plan-starts-with-a-tough-premise-repeal-all-of-obamacare/.

3. Eric M. Patashnik, *Reforms at Risk: What Happens after Major Policy Changes Are Enacted* (Princeton, NJ: Princeton University Press, 2008).

4. This form of intergovernmental negotiation is captured in Robert Agranoff and Michael McGuire, "Another Look at Bargaining and Negotiation in Intergovernmental Management," *Journal of Public Administration Research and Theory* 14, no. 4 (2004): 495–512.

5. Throughout this book, terms such as *ideology* and *ideological* do not refer to a Marxist perspective, according to which "ideology" is the opposite of objective, scientific truth and a pure distortion of reality. Instead, in this book, ideology simply refers to relatively systematic world-views. On the concept of ideology, see Sheri Berman, "Understanding the Origins of Ideology: The Case of European Social Democracy," in *Ideas and Politics in Social Science Research,* ed. Daniel Béland and Robert Henry Cox (New York: Oxford University Press, 2011), 105–126; Michael Freeden, *Ideology: A Very Short Introduction* (Oxford, UK: Oxford University Press, 2003).

6. Heather Gerken and Jessica Bulman-Pozen, "Uncooperative Federalism," *Yale Law Journal* 118, no. 7 (2009): 1256–1310.

7. David Brian Robertson, "Madison's Opponents and Constitutional Design," *American Political Science Review* 99, no. 2 (2005): 226.

8. David Brian Robertson, *Federalism and the Making of America* (London: Routledge, 2012).

9. Terry Moe, "The Politics of Bureaucratic Structure," in *Can the Government Govern?* ed. John E. Chubb and Paul E. Peterson (Washington, DC: Brookings Institution Press, 1989), 276.

10. *McCulloch v. Maryland,* 17 U.S. 316 (1819).

11. Robertson, *Federalism and the Making of America,* 129–148.

12. Alan Brinkley, "Re-legitimizing Government," in *New Federalist Papers,* ed. Alan Brinkley, Nelson W. Polsby, and Kathleen M. Sullivan (New York: Norton, 1997), 125–126.

13. Daniel Béland and Alex Waddan, *The Politics of Policy Change* (Washington, DC: Georgetown University Press, 2012).

14. Paul Pierson, *Politics in Time: History, Institutions, and Social Analysis* (Princeton, NJ: Princeton University Press, 2004). See also Moe, "Politics of Bureaucratic Structure."

15. Sheryl Gay Stolberg and Robert Pear, "Obama Signs Health Care Overhaul into Law, with a Flourish," *New York Times,* March 24, 2010, accessed April 27, 2014, http://www.nytimes.com /2010/03/24/health/policy/24health.html?_r=0.

16. Sven Steinmo and Jon Watts, "It's the Institutions, Stupid! Why Comprehensive National Health Insurance Always Fails in America," *Journal of Health Policy, Politics, and Law* 20, no. 2 (1995): 329–372.

17. Jeffrey Pressman and Aaron Wildavsky, *Implementation,* 2nd ed. (Berkeley: University of California Press, 1979), 110. See also Eugene Bardach, *The Implementation Game: What Happens after a Bill Becomes a Law* (Cambridge: Massachusetts Institute of Technology Press, 1977); Martha Derthick, *New Towns in-Town* (Washington, DC: Urban Institute, 1972).

18. Eric M. Patashnik, "After the Public Interest Prevails: The Political Sustainability of Policy Reform," *Governance* 16, no. 2 (2003): 226.

19. See Kimberly Krawiec, "Don't 'Screw Joe the Plummer': The Sausage Making of Financial Reform," *Arizona Law Review* 55 (2013): 53–103. Consider the Dodd-Frank reforms of financial regulation after the economic crisis of 2008. The so-called Volcker Rule, one of the reform's most notable provisions for limiting risky activity, gave substantial discretion to banking regulators to create policy as they saw fit. Because these regulators were obligated to open their procedures to notice-and-comment proceedings by interested parties, the process was ripe for political contestation from the opponents of financial reform, who were disproportionately represented in notice-and-comment proceedings and meetings with regulators.

20. The scholarly literature tends not to treat these two processes together, but an increasing number of political scientists and legal scholars have begun to challenge this trend. See Gerken and Bulman-Pozen, "Uncooperative Federalism"; Jessica Bulman-Pozen, "Partisan Federalism," *Harvard Law Review* 127 (Winter 2014): 1017–1145; John Dinan, "The State of American Federal-

ism 2007–2008: Resurgent State Influence in the National Policy Process and Continued State Policy Innovation," *Publius: The Journal of Federalism* 38, no. 3 (2008): 381–415.

21. Paul Pierson, "Fragmented Welfare States: Federal Institutions and the Development of Social Policy," *Governance* 8, no. 4 (October 1995): 449–478.

22. Jacob S. Hacker, "Privatizing Risk without Privatizing the Welfare State: The Hidden Politics of Social Policy Retrenchment in the United States," *American Political Science Review* 98, no. 2 (2004): 243–260; James Mahoney and Kathleen Thelen, "A Theory of Gradual Institutional Change," in *Explaining Institutional Change: Ambiguity, Agency, and Power*, ed. James Mahoney and Kathleen Thelen (New York: Cambridge University Press, 2010), 1–37; Philip Rocco and Chloe Thurston, "From Metaphors to Measures: Observable Indicators of Gradual Institutional Change," *Journal of Public Policy* 34, no. 1 (2014): 35–62.

23. Gerken and Bulman-Pozen, "Uncooperative Federalism."

24. Bulman-Pozen, "Partisan Federalism."

25. Paul E. Peterson, Barry G. Rabe, and Kenneth K. Wong, *When Federalism Works* (Washington, DC: Brookings Institution Press, 1986): 191–215.

26. Ibid.

27. Frank J. Thompson and Courtney Burke, "Federalism by Waiver: Medicaid and the Transformation of Long-Term Care," *Publius: The Journal of Federalism* 39, no. 1 (2009): 22–46.

28. Federal official, interview by Philip Rocco, February 15, 2013.

29. Ibid.

30. Centers for Medicare and Medicaid Services, "Proposed Rule CMS-9989-P: Establishment of Exchanges and Qualified Health Plans," accessed April 27, 2014, http://www.gpo.gov/fdsys/pkg/FR-2011-07-15/pdf/2011-17610.pdf.

31. Rocco interview, February 15, 2013.

32. Centers for Medicare and Medicaid Services, "Final Rule CMS-9989-F: Establishment of Exchanges and Qualified Health Plans—Exchange Standards for Employers," accessed April 27, 2014, http://www.gpo.gov/fdsys/pkg/FR-2011-07-15/pdf/2011-17610.pdf.

33. David Brian Robertson, "The Bias of American Federalism: The Limits of Welfare-State Development in the Progressive Era," *Journal of Policy History* 1, no. 3 (1989): 261–291; Jeffrey L. Pressman and Aaron Wildavsky, *Implementation* (Berkeley: University of California Press, 1973); John D. Donahue, *Disunited States* (New York: BasicBooks, 1997).

34. Erin Ryan, "Negotiating Federalism," *Boston Law Review* 52, no. 1 (2011): 1–136.

35. Robert Agranoff and Michael McGuire, *Collaborative Public Management: New Strategies for Local Governments* (Washington, DC: Georgetown University Press, 2004).

36. Martha Derthick, *Agency under Stress: The Social Security Administration in American Government* (Washington, DC: Brookings Institution Press, 1990).

37. Michael J. Scicchitano and David M. Hedge, "From Coercion to Partnership in Federal Partial Preemption: SMCRA, RCRA, and OSH Act," *Publius: The Journal of Federalism* 23, no. 4 (1993): 107–121.

38. Peter H. Schuck, "Taking Immigration Federalism Seriously," *University of Chicago Legal Forum* (2007): 57.

39. Scicchitano and Hedge, "From Coercion to Partnership in Federal Partial Preemption."

40. James E. Monogan, "The Politics of Immigrant Policy in the 50 US States, 2005–2011," *Journal of Public Policy* 33, no. 1 (2013): 35–64.

41. Paul L. Posner, *The Politics of Unfunded Mandates: Whither Federalism?* (Washington, DC: Georgetown University Press, 1998).

42. John Dinan, "Implementing Health Reform: Intergovernmental Bargaining and the Affordable Care Act," *Publius: The Journal of Federalism* 44, no. 3 (2014): 399–425.

43. Agranoff and McGuire, "Another Look at Bargaining and Negotiating in Intergovernmental Management," 495–512.

44. A thorough typology of grants can be found in Sean C. Nicholson-Crotty, "Goal Conflict and Fund Diversion in Federal Grants to the States," *American Journal of Political Science* 48, no. 1 (2004): 110–122.

45. PEW Center for the States, Fiscal Federal Initiative, "Federal Grants Provide $1 out of Every $3 in State Revenues after the Great Recession," accessed April 27, 2014, http://www.pewstates .org/news-room/press-releases/federal-grants-provide-1-out-of-every-3-in-state-revenues-after -the-great-recession-85899506260.

46. Circulars from the Office of Management and Budget (OMB) are especially telling on this point. See, for example, White House Office of Management and Budget, "Uniform Administrative Requirements for Grants and Agreements with Institutions of Higher Education, Hospitals, and Other Non-Profit Organizations, Circular A11," accessed April 27, 2014, http://www .whitehouse.gov/omb/circulars_a110/.

47. James L. Sundquist and David W. Davis, *Making Federalism Work* (Washington, DC: Brookings Institution Press, 1969).

48. Hugh Davis Graham, *The Uncertain Triumph: Federal Education Policy in the Kennedy and Johnson Years* (Chapel Hill: University of North Carolina Press, 2011). As Graham puts it, "When Title I was implemented, it produced not *a* Title I program, but something more like 30,000 separate and different Title I programs" (204–205). Over time, however, increased funds for federal enforcement activities allowed for more rigorous application procedures associated with grant renewal as well as additional monitoring of state and local activity. Though the grant bargaining conditions changed, bargaining itself did not disappear. Because states' views continued to conflict with federal policy prescriptions, they continued to push federal education officials to loosen the requirements for receiving federal grants.

49. Advisory Commission on Intergovernmental Relations (ACIR), Federal Statutory Preemption of State and Local Authority: History, Inventory, and Issues, A-121 (Washington, DC: ACIR, 1992).

50. Scicchitano and Hedge, "From Coercion to Partnership in Federal Partial Preemption."

51. ACIR, Federal Statutory Preemption of State and Local Authority.

52. George C. Eads and Michael Fix, eds., *The Reagan Regulatory Strategy: An Assessment* (Washington, DC: Urban Institute, 1984).

53. Thomas Gais and James Fossett, "Federalism and the Executive Branch," in *The Executive Branch*, ed. Joel Aberbach and Mark Peterson (New York: Oxford University Press, 2005), 486–522.

54. Frank J. Thompson and Courtney Burke, "Executive Federalism and Medicaid Demonstration Waivers: Implications for Policy and Democratic Process," *Journal of Health Politics, Policy, and Law* 32, no. 6 (2007): 971–1004; Frank J. Thompson, *Medicaid Politics: Federalism, Policy Durability, and Health Reform* (Washington, DC: Georgetown University Press, 2012).

55. Carol S. Weissert and William G. Weissert, *Governing Health: The Politics of Health Policy* (Baltimore, MD: Johns Hopkins University Press, 2008).

56. Thompson and Burke, "Executive Federalism and Medicaid Demonstration Waivers," 971–1004.

57. Saundra K. Schneider, "Medicaid Section 1115 Waivers: Shifting Health Care Reform to the States," *Publius: The Journal of Federalism* 27, no. 2 (1997): 89–109.

58. Thompson, *Medicaid Politics.*

59. Megan Mullin and Dorothy M. Daley, "Working with the State: Exploring Interagency Collaboration within a Federalism System," *Journal of Public Administration Research and Theory* 20, no. 4 (2010): 757-778; Pierson, "Fragmented Welfare States," 449-478.

60. Anne Marie Cammisa, *Governments as Interest Groups: Intergovernmental Lobbying and the Federal System* (Westport, CT: Greenwood, 1995).

61. Amy McKay and Susan Webb Yackee, "Interest Group Competition on Federal Agency Rules," *American Politics Research* 35, no. 3 (2007): 336-357; Jason Webb Yackee and Susan Webb Yackee, "A Bias towards Business? Assessing Interest Group Influence on the US Bureaucracy," *Journal of Politics* 68, no. 1 (2006): 128-139; Kevin M. Esterling, "Does the Federal Government Learn from the States? Medicaid and the Limits of Expertise in the Intergovernmental Lobby," *Publius: The Journal of Federalism* 39, no. 1 (2009): 1-21.

62. Derthick, *Agency under Stress,* 22-32.

63. Ibid.

64. John Dinan, "Contemporary Assertions of State Sovereignty and the Safeguards of American Federalism," *Albany Law Review* 74, no. 4 (2011): 1635-1667; Gerken and Bulman-Pozen, "Uncooperative Federalism."

65. Andrew Koppelman, *The Tough Luck Constitution and the Assault on Healthcare Reform* (New York: Oxford University Press, 2013).

66. Heritage Foundation Blog, "List of States Suing over Obamacare," January 17, 2011, accessed April 27, 2014, http://blog.heritage.org/2011/01/17/list-of-states-suing-over-obamacare/.

67. Koppelman, *Tough Luck Constitution.*

68. Jonathan Oberlander, "The Future of Obamacare," *New England Journal of Medicine* 367, no. 23 (2012): 2165-2167.

69. Sean Beienburg, "Contesting the US Constitution through State Amendments: The 2011 and 2012 Elections," *Political Science Quarterly* 129, no. 1 (2014): 55-85; Daniel Béland, Philip Rocco, and Alex Waddan, "Implementing Health Care Reform in the United States: Intergovernmental Politics and the Dilemmas of Institutional Design," *Health Policy* 116 (Spring 2014): 142-143.

70. Sarah A. Binder, *Stalemate: Causes and Consequences of Legislative Gridlock* (Washington, DC: Brookings Institution Press, 2003).

71. Dinan, "Contemporary Assertions of State Sovereignty and the Safeguards of American Federalism."

72. Johannes Lindvall, "Politics and Policies in Two Economic Crises: The Nordic Countries," in *Coping with Crisis,* ed. Nancy Bermeo and Jonas Pontusson (New York: Russell Sage Foundation, 2012): 233-260.

73. James Roger Sharp, *American Politics in the Early Republic: The New Nation in Crisis* (New Haven, CT: Yale University Press, 1993).

74. Erin N. Waltenburg and Bill Swinford, *Litigating Federalism: The States before the US Supreme Court* (Westport, CT: Greenwood, 1999).

75. Paul Nolette, "State Litigation during the Obama Administration: Diverging Agendas in an Era of Polarized Politics," *Publius: The Journal of Federalism* 44, no. 3 (2014): 451-473.

76. Denise Scheberle, *Federalism and Environmental Policy: Trust and the Politics of Implementation* (Washington, DC: Georgetown University Press, 2004).

77. Nolette, "State Litigation during the Obama Administration."

78. Dinan, "Contemporary Assertions of State Sovereignty and the Safeguards of American Federalism."

79. Ibid.

80. Priscilla M. Regan and Christopher J. Deering, "State Opposition to REAL ID," *Publius: The Journal of Federalism* 39, no. 3 (2009): 476–505.

81. Ibid.

82. Scicchitano and Hedge, "From Coercion to Partnership in Federal Partial Preemption."

83. Samuel Hutchison Beer, *To Make a Nation: The Rediscovery of American Federalism* (Cambridge, MA: Harvard University Press, 1993).

84. J. Mitchell Pickerill and Cornell W. Clayton, "The Rehnquist Court and the Political Dynamics of Federalism," *Perspectives on Politics* 2, no. 2 (2004): 233–248.

85. Timothy J. Conlan, *From New Federalism to Devolution: Twenty-Five Years of Intergovernmental Reform* (Washington, DC: Brookings Institution Press, 1998).

86. Paul Manna, "Control, Persuasion, and Educational Accountability: Implementing the No Child Left Behind Act," *Educational Policy* 20, no. 3 (2006): 471–494.

87. Dinan, "Contemporary Assertions of State Sovereignty and the Safeguards of American Federalism"; Gerken and Bulman-Pozen, "Uncooperative Federalism."

88. Because not all political opponents have the same resources to engage in political battles, this might be another source of variation to exploit. However, because even political actors with sizable financial reserves and organizational capacity must do battle in the institutional contexts we lay out here, we exclude variation in resources from our main argument.

89. Peterson, Rabe, and Wong, *When Federalism Works.*

90. Paul Pierson, *Dismantling the Welfare State? Reagan, Thatcher, and the Politics of Retrenchment* (New York: Cambridge University Press, 1994); Margaret Weir, Ann Shola Orloff, and Theda Skocpol, eds., *The Politics of Social Policy in the United States* (Princeton, NJ: Princeton University Press, 1988).

91. Denise Scheberle, "The Evolving Matrix of Environmental Federalism and Intergovernmental Relationships," *Publius: The Journal of Federalism* 35, no. 1 (2005): 69–86.

92. Barbara Warner and Jennifer Shapiro, "Fractured, Fragmented Federalism: A Study in Fracking Regulatory Policy," *Publius: The Journal of Federalism* 43, no. 3 (2013): 474–496.

93. Erin Ryan, "Negotiating Federalism," *Boston Law Review* 52, no. 1 (2011): 1–136.

94. Gerken and Bulman-Pozen, "Uncooperative Federalism."

95. Ibid.

96. Pierson, "Fragmented Welfare States."

97. Abbe R. Gluck, "Intrastatutory Federalism and Statutory Interpretation: State Implementation of Federal Law in Health Reform and Beyond," *Yale Law Journal* 121 (2011): 534–621.

98. Michael J. Scicchitano, David M. Hedge, and Patricia Metz, "The States and Deregulation: The Case of Surface Mining," *Review of Policy Research* 9, no. 1 (1989): 120–131.

99. Scicchitano and Hedge, "From Coercion to Partnership in Federal Partial Preemption."

100. Ellen M. Immergut, "Institutions, Veto Points, and Policy Results: A Comparative Analysis of Health Care," *Journal of Public Policy* 10, no. 4 (1990): 391–416.

101. William R. Lowry, *The Dimensions of Federalism: State Governments and Pollution Control Policies* (Durham, NC: Duke University Press, 1996).

102. Gerken and Bulman-Pozen, "Uncooperative Federalism."

103. John L. Campbell, *Institutional Change and Globalization* (Princeton, NJ: Princeton University Press, 2004), 96. For evidence of how this process shaped the political opportunities of opponents to Medicare, see Kimberly J. Morgan and Andrea Louise Campbell, *The Delegated Welfare State: Medicare, Markets, and the Governance of Social Policy* (New York: Oxford University Press, 2011).

104. Jeffrey A. Brook, "Measuring Issue Salience," *American Journal of Political Science* 44, no. 1 (2000): 66–83.

105. Robert S. Erikson, Michael B. MacKuen, and James A. Stimson, *The Macro Polity* (New York: Cambridge University Press, 2002).

106. Chris Koski, "Greening America's Skylines: The Diffusion of Low-Salience Policies," *Policy Studies Journal* 38, no. 1 (2010): 93–117.

107. Richard L. Cole, John Kincaid, and Andrew Parkin, "Public Opinion on Federalism in the United States and Canada in 2002: The Aftermath of Terrorism," *Publius: The Journal of Federalism* 32, no. 4 (2002): 123–148.

108. Peter Eisinger, "Imperfect Federalism: The Intergovernmental Partnership for Homeland Security," *Public Administration Review* 66, no. 4 (2006): 537–545.

109. Bryan Shelly, "Rebels and Their Causes: State Resistance to No Child Left Behind," *Publius: The Journal of Federalism* 38, no. 3 (2008): 444–468.

110. For examples of excellent studies on the ACA that rely on single reforms, see Simon F. Haeder and David L. Weimer, "You Can't Make Me Do It: State Implementation of Insurance Exchanges under the Affordable Care Act," *Public Administration Review* 73, no. 1 (2013): 34–47; Elizabeth Rigby and Jake Haselswerdt, "Hybrid Federalism, Partisan Politics, and Early Implementation of State Health Insurance Exchanges," *Publius: The Journal of Federalism* 43, no. 3 (2013): 368–391; Lawrence R. Jacobs and Timothy Callaghan, "Why States Expand Medicaid: Party, Resources, and History," *Journal of Health Politics, Policy, and Law* 38, no. 5 (2013): 1023–1050.

111. Here we combine cross-case analysis with in-case comparisons, as discussed in Alexander L. George and Andrew Bennett, *Case Studies and Theory Development in the Social Sciences* (Cambridge: Massachusetts Institute of Technology Press, 2005), 151–180.

112. Daniel Béland, "Reconsidering Policy Feedback: How Policies Affect Politics," *Administration and Society* 42, no. 5 (2010): 568–590.

2. UNCERTAIN VICTORY

1. Sheryl Gay Stolberg and Robert Pear, "Obama Signs Health Care Overhaul Bill, with a Flourish," *New York Times,* March 23, 2010.

2. Mitch McConnell, "Obamacare Will Be the Focus of 2014 Midterms," *Unedited Politics,* May 19, 2013, accessed November 12, 2014, http://uneditedpolitics.com/mitch-mcconnell-on-meet-the-press-obamacare-will-be-focus-of-2014-midterm-51913/.

3. Max Baucus made this statement at a Senate Budget Committee hearing in April 2013 when expressing his anxiety to Kathleen Sebelius, secretary of Health and Human Services, that there was not enough information in the public domain about how the new law would work. Tom Kertscher, "In Context: Obamacare 'Train Wreck,'" Politifact.com, August 6, 2013, accessed November 14, 2014, www.politifact.com/wisconsin/article/2013aug/06/context-obama-train-wreck/.

4. Deidre Walsh, "House Passes 50th Bill to Undo Obamacare," CNN Political Ticker, March 5, 2014, accessed November 13, 2014, http://politicalticker.blogs.cnn.com/2014/03/05/house-passes-50th-bill-to-undo-obamacare/.

5. Lawrence R. Jacobs and Theda Skocpol, *Health Care Reform and American Politics: What Everyone Needs to Know* (New York: Oxford University Press, 2010).

6. Eric M. Patashnik and Julian E. Zelizer, "The Struggle to Remake Politics: Liberal Reform and the Limits of Policy Feedback in the Contemporary American State," *Perspectives on Politics* 11, no. 4 (2013): 1073.

7. Elizabeth Rigby, Jennifer Hayes Clark, and Stacey Pelika, "Party Politics and the Enactment of 'Obamacare': A Policy-Centered Analysis of Minority Party Involvement," *Journal of Health Politics, Policy, and Law* 39, no. 1 (2014): 59.

8. Scott Greer, "The States' Role under the Patient Protection and Affordable Care Act," *Journal of Health Politics, Policy, and Law* 36, no. 3 (2011): 471.

9. Jonathon Cohn, "How They Did It: The Inside Account of Health Care Reform's Triumph," *New Republic,* May 21, 2010, accessed November 16, 2014, http://www.newrepublic.com/article /75077/how-they-did-it.

10. Lawrence Jacobs and Theda Skocpol, "Hard-Fought Legacy: Obama, Congressional Democrats, and the Struggle for Comprehensive Health Care Reform," in *Reaching for a New Deal: Ambitious Governance, Economic Meltdown, and Polarized Politics in Obama's First Two Years,* ed. Theda Skocpol and Lawrence Jacobs (New York: Russell Sage Foundation, 2011), 59.

11. Ezekiel Emmanuel, *Reinventing American Health Care: How the Affordable Health Care Act Will Improve Our Terribly Complex, Blatantly Unjust, Outrageously Expensive, Grossly Inefficient, Error-Prone System* (New York: PublicAffairs, 2014), 160.

12. Jacob Hacker, "Why Reform Happened," *Journal of Health Politics, Policy, and Law* 36, no. 3 (2011): 437–441.

13. Rhodes Cook, "Not Your Father's Democratic Congress," Sabato's Crystal Ball, February 19, 2009, accessed November 14, 2014, http://www.centerforpolitics.org/crystalball/articles/frc 2009021901/.

14. Mark Peterson, "It Was a Different Time: Obama and the Unique Opportunity for Health Care Reform," *Journal of Health Politics, Policy, and Law* 36, no. 3 (2011): 431.

15. Jackie Calmes, "Clinton's Health Defeat Sways Obama's Tactics," *New York Times,* September 5, 2009.

16. Michael Doonan and Katherine Tull, "Health Care Reform in Massachusetts: Implementation of Coverage Expansions and a Health Insurance Mandate," *Millbank Quarterly* 88, no. 1 (2010): 54–80.

17. Pam Belluck and Katie Zezima, "Massachusetts Legislation on Insurance Becomes Law," *New York Times,* April 13, 2006.

18. Ibid. The authors of the *New York Times* piece also commented, "Mr. Romney is considering running for president in 2008, and the success of the bipartisan health care plan could become a major selling point of his candidacy."

19. Edmund F. Haislmaier and Nina Owcharenko, "The Massachusetts Approach: A New Way to Restructure State Health Insurance Markets and Public Programs," *Health Affairs* 25, no. 6 (2006): 1581.

20. Ibid.

21. Doonan and Tull, "Health Care Reform in Massachusetts." For an analysis of the state's previous moves to regulate insurers there, see R. Curtis, S. Lewis, K. Haugh, and R. Forland, "Health Insurance Reform in the Small-Group Market," *Health Affairs* 18, no. 3 (1999): 151–160.

22. Paul Starr, *Remedy and Reaction: The Peculiar American Struggle over Health Care Reform* (New Haven, CT: Yale University Press, 2011), 14.

23. Ceci Connolly, "How We Got There," in *Landmark: The Inside Story of America's New Health-Care Law and What It Means for Us All,* ed. *Washington Post* Staff (New York: Public Affairs, 2010).

24. Robert Pear and Sheryl Gay Stolberg, "Obama Says He Is Open to Altering Health Plan," *New York Times,* March 5, 2009, accessed November 12, 2014, http://www.nytimes.com /2009/03/06/us/politics/06web-health.html.

25. Jeff Zeleny, "Obama: 'Stars Are Aligned' This Year for Health Care," *New York Times*, May 13, 2009, accessed November 10, 2014, http://thecaucus.blogs.nytimes.com/2009/05/13/obama -stars-are-aligned-this-year-for-health-care/.

26. Jacobs and Skocpol, *Health Care Reform and American Politics*, 85.

27. Emily Smith, "Timeline of the Health Care Law," CNN, June 28, 2012, accessed November 10, 2014, http://edition.cnn.com/2012/06/28/politics/supreme-court-health-timeline/.

28. David Herszenhorn, "Senate Committee Approves Health Care Bill," *New York Times*, July 15, 2009, accessed November 17, 2014, http://thecaucus.blogs.nytimes.com/2009/07/15/senate -committee-approves-health-care-bill/?_r=0.

29. David Herszenhorn and Robert Pear, "Health Policy Is Carved Out at a Table for Six," *New York Times*, July 28, 2009, A1.

30. Katharine Seelye, "The Gang of Six Will Talk at 9," *New York Times*, August 19, 2009, accessed November 17, 2014, http://prescriptions.blogs.nytimes.com/2009/08/19/the-gang-of-six -will-talk-at-9/.

31. James Brasfield, "The Politics of Ideas: Where Did the Public Option Come from and Where Is It Going?" *Journal of Health Politics, Policy, and Law* 36, no. 3 (2011): 455–459.

32. Democratic congressional staffer, interview with Daniel Béland, August 2010.

33. Shana Rose, *Financing Medicaid: Federalism and the Growth of American Health Care's Safety Net* (Ann Arbor: University of Michigan Press, 2013), 230–234.

34. Michael Sparer, "Federalism and the Patient Protection and Affordable Care Act of 2010: The Founding Fathers Would Not Be Surprised," *Journal of Health Politics, Policy, and Law* 36, no. 3 (2011): 463.

35. Greg Sargent, "Senate Documents and Interviews Undercut 'Bombshell' Lawsuit against Obamacare," *Washington Post*, July 29, 2014, accessed November 20, 2014, http://www.washington post.com/blogs/plum-line/wp/2014/07/29/senate-documents-and-interviews-undercut-bomb shell-lawsuit-against-obamacare/. The SFC's bill did not specifically mention the notion of the federal government taking over the state's responsibility for setting up an exchange because it implied states would have to set up their own arrangements. The federally run exchange was developed in the Senate Health, Education, Labor, and Pensions Committee and found its way into the merged Senate bill. On the absence of penalties, see Theda Skocpol and Larry Jacobs, "Progressive Federalism and the Contested Implementation of Obama's Health Reform," in *The Politics of Major Policy Reform in Postwar America*, ed. Jeffery A. Jenkins and Sidney M. Milkis (New York: Cambridge University Press, 2014), 157–178.

36. Karen Davis, Stuart Guterman, Sara Collins, Kristof Stremikis, Sheila Rustgi, and Rachel Nuzum, "Starting on the Path to a High-Performance Health System: Analysis of Health System Reform Provisions of Reform Bills in the House of Representatives and Senate," Commonwealth Fund, last modified December 4, 2009, accessed November 16, 2014, http://www.commonwealth fund.org/publications/fund-reports/2009/nov/starting-on-the-path-to-a-high-performance -health-system.

37. Timothy Jost, transcript from debate organized by the Alliance for Health Reform, "Health Insurance Exchanges: House or Senate Style?" January 8, 2010, accessed November 16, 2014, www .allhealth.org/briefingmaterials/HealthInsuranceExchangesTranscript-FINAL-1.

38. Ibid.

39. Kaiser Family Foundation, "President-Elect Barack Obama's Campaign Positions on Health Care," 2013, accessed November 14, 2014, http://kaiserfamilyfoundation.files.wordpress .com/2013/01/obama_campaign_position_on_health_care.pdf.

40. Sparer, "Federalism and the Patient Protection and Affordable Care Act of 2010." Accord-

ing to Senator Olympia Snowe, members of the Gang of Six did negotiate seriously and were especially sensitive to the concerns of governors. Tom Daschle with David Nather, *Getting It Done: How Obama and Congress Finally Broke the Stalemate to Make Way for Health Care Reform* (New York: Thomas Dunne Books, 2010), 194. On the role of centrist Democrats, see Skocpol and Jacobs, "Progressive Federalism and the Contested Implementation of Obama's Health Reform."

41. Wendy Stein, "MLR: The Controversial Calculation Makes Its Appearance in the Health Care Reform Debate," *ABA Health* 6, no. 7 (2010), accessed November 14, 2014, https://www .americanbar.org/newsletter/publications/aba_health_esource_home/Stein.html.

42. John D. Rockefeller IV to H. Edward Hanway, letter, November 2, 2009, accessed November 17, 2014, http://www.commerce.senate.gov/public/?a=Files.Serve&File_id=aae8e105–4752 –459d-9bc5-d0b68576cb50.

43. Kate Pickert, "Forcing Insurers to Spend Enough on Health Care," *Time*, December 22, 2009, accessed November 2, 2014, http://www.time.com/time/nation/article/0,8599,1949390,00.html.

44. Stein, "MLR."

45. Julie Appleby, "Democrats Move to Regulate How Insurers Spend Customers' Money," *Kaiser Health News*, last modified December 24, 2009, accessed November 14, 2014, http://kaiser healthnews.org/news/insurers/.

46. Jacobs and Skocpol, *Health Care Reform and American Politics*, 101.

47. Sheryl Gay Stolberg and David Herszenhorn, "Obama Weighs Paring Goals for Health Bill," *New York Times*, January 20, 2010. Some liberals, unsatisfied with the compromises made through 2009, shared this sentiment. See Robert Kuttner, *A Presidency in Peril: The Inside Story of Obama's Promise, Wall Street's Power, and the Struggle to Control Our Economic Future* (White River Junction, VT: Chelsea Green, 2010), 233.

48. Fred Barnes, "The Health Care Bill Is Dead," *Weekly Standard*, January 10, 2010, accessed November 14, 2014, http://www.weeklystandard.com/blogs/health-care-bill-dead.

49. Jacobs and Skocpol, *Health Care Reform and American Politics*, 111–119.

50. Daschle with Nather, *Getting It Done*, 234. Daschle was former Senate majority leader and Democratic minority leader until he was defeated in the 2004 election. He was an early, high-profile supporter of Barack Obama's campaign for the presidency and was nominated to serve as secretary of Health and Human Services by the new president. He withdrew his name from consideration when a scandal blew up over unpaid taxes.

51. Carrie Budoff Brown, "Nelson: National Exchange a Deal Breaker," *Politico*, January 25, 2010, accessed November 1, 2014, http://www.politico.com/livepulse/0110/Nelson_National _exchange_a_dealbreaker.html. Nelson in fact made this statement after Scott Brown's election, meaning that the Democrats had already lost their sixty votes.

52. Jacobs and Skocpol, *Health Care Reform and American Politics*, 161.

53. E. J. Dionne, "The Alternative Is Catastrophe," *New Republic*, January 11, 2010, accessed November 3, 2014, www.newrepublic.com/article/politics/the-alternative-catastrophe.

54. Jacobs and Skocpol, *Health Care Reform and American Politics*, 161.

55. Robert Pear, "U.S. Officials Brace for Huge Task of Operating Health Exchanges," *New York Times*, August 5, 2012, A17.

56. Jacobs and Skocpol, *Health Care Reform and American Politics*, 164.

57. Timothy Jost, "Implementation and Enforcement of Health Care Reform—Federal versus State Government," *New England Journal of Medicine*, January 14, 2010, accessed October 28, 2014, www.nejm.org/doi/full/10.1056/NEJMp0911636.

58. For a detailed description of the deal making involved, see Jacobs and Skocpol, *Health Care Reform and American Politics*, 66–75.

59. Haynes Johnson and David Broder, *The System: The American Way of Politics at Breaking Point* (Boston: Little, Brown, 1997), 234.

60. Andrea Louise Campbell, *How Policies Make Citizens: Senior Political Activism and the American Welfare State* (Princeton, NJ: Princeton University Press, 2005).

61. Theda Skocpol, *Boomerang: Health Care Reform and the Turn against Government* (New York: Norton, 1997), 4–5.

62. Paul Starr, "What Happened to Health Care Reform?" *American Prospect* 20 (1995): 20.

63. Stanley Greenberg, *Middle-Class Dreams: The Politics and Power of the New American Majority* (New Haven, CT: Yale University Press, 1995), 308.

64. Jill Quadagno, "Right Wing Conspiracy? Socialist Plot? The Origins of the Patient Protection and Affordable Care Act," *Journal of Health Politics, Policy, and Law* 39, no. 1 (2014): 33–56.

65. Stuart Butler, "Don't Blame Heritage for Obamacare Mandate," *USA Today*, February 6, 2012, accessed October 30, 2014, http://usatoday30.usatoday.com/news/opinion/forum/story /2012–02–03/health-individual-mandate-reform-heritage/52951140/1.

66. "Interview with Minority Leader John Boehner," Real Clear Politics, January 20, 2010, accessed November 3, 2014, http://www.realclearpolitics.com/articles/2010/01/20/interview_with _minority_leader_john_boehner_99997.html.

67. Carl Hulse and Adam Nagourney, "Senate GOP Leader Finds Weapon in Unity," *New York Times*, March 17, 2010, A13.

68. Ibid.

69. Patashnik and Zelizer, "The Struggle to Remake Politics," 1077.

70. Jacob Hacker and Paul Pierson, "After the 'Master Theory': Downs, Schattschneider, and the Rebirth of Policy-Focused Analysis," May 2014, accessed October 28, 2014, www.maxpo.eu /Downloads/Paper_Pierson.pdf. On "policy as prize" see Rigby et al., "Party Politics and the Enactment of 'Obamacare,'" 59.

71. Kathleen Bawn, Martin Cohen, David Karol, Seth Masket, Hans Noel, and John Zaller, "A Theory of Political Parties: Groups, Policy Demands, and Nominations in American Politics," *Perspectives on Politics* 10, no. 3 (2012): 571–597.

72. Ian Urbina, "Beyond Beltway, Health Debate Turns Hostile," *New York Times*, August 8, 2009, A1. For an analysis that emphasizes the well-organized and well-financed groups that orchestrated the protests, see Starr, *Remedy and Reaction*, 214–216. On the rise of the Tea Party, see Theda Skocpol and Vanessa Williamson, *The Tea Party and the Remaking of Republican Conservatism* (New York: Oxford University Press, 2012).

73. Carl Hulse, "Conservative Group Targets Gang of Six Republicans," *New York Times*, August 20, 2009, accessed October 29, 2014, http://prescriptions.blogs.nytimes.com/2009/08/20 /conservative-group-targets-gang-of-6-republicans.

74. Robert Pear and David Herszenhorn, "Republican's Vote Lifts a Health Bill, but Hurdles Remain," *New York Times*, October 14, 2009, A1. According to Jonathon Cohn's account, some of Grassley's staffers "joined Baucus on a quixotic hunt for Republicans willing to support reform on the floor," but in the end the pressure to make a public stand against reform was too much, especially when "Iowa conservatives began threatening to back a primary challenge if Grassley ever voted for health reform." By that time Grassley was echoing the "'death panels' language of Sarah Palin as he told a group of constituents: 'We should not have a government program that determines if you're going to pull the plug on grandma.'" Cohn, "How They Did It: The Inside Account of Health Care Reform's Triumph."

75. For revealing details of how NFIB and HIAA developed their strategies in 1993, see Johnson and Broder, *System*, 206–224.

76. Daschle with Nather, *Getting It Done*, 83–84.

77. Matthew J. Lebo and Andrew J. O'Geen, "The President's Role in the Partisan Congressional Arena," *Journal of Politics* 73, no. 3 (2011): 718–734.

78. Daniel Béland, Philip Rocco, and Alex Waddan, "Implementing Health Reform in the United States: The Dilemmas of Institutional Design," *Health Policy* 116, no. 1 (2014): 51–60.

79. Robert Rich and William White, "Health Care Policy and the American States: Issues of Federalism," in *Health Policy, Federalism, and the American States*, ed. Robert Rich and William White (Washington, DC: Urban Institute Press, 1996), 6.

80. US Bureau of the Census, "Health Insurance Historical Tables," Table HIB-4. In *Health Insurance Coverage Status and Type of Coverage by State, All People: 1999 to 2012*, accessed November 2, 2014, http://www.census.gov/hhes/www/hlthins/data/historical/HIB_tables.html.

81. National Association of Insurance Commissioners, *Patient Protection and Affordable Care Act: Section by Section Analysis* (Washington, DC: NAIC, 2011).

82. American Legislative Exchange Council, "About ALEC's Freedom of Choice in Health Care Act," accessed November 2, 2014, http://www.alec.org/initiatives/health-care-freedom -initiative/about-alecs-freedom-of-choice-in-health-care-act/.

83. National Council of State Legislatures, *State Laws and Actions Challenging Certain Health Reforms*, last modified November 7, 2014, accessed October 24, 2014, http://www.ncsl.org/research /health/state-laws-and-actions-challenging-ppaca.aspx.

84. Karen Hansen, "A GOP Wave Washed over State Legislatures on Election Day," National Council of State Legislatures, last modified December 2010, accessed October 20, 2014, http:// www.ncsl.org/research/elections-and-campaigns/red-tide.aspx.

85. Robert Saldin, "Healthcare Reform: A Prescription for the 2010 Republican Landslide?" *Forum* 8, no. 4 (2010).

86. Henry Aaron, "Here to Stay: Beyond the Rough Launch of the ACA," *New England Journal of Medicine* 370 (2014): 2257–2259.

87. Wendy Mariner, Leonard Glantz, and George Annas, "Reframing Federalism: The Affordable Care Act (and Broccoli) in the Supreme Court," *New England Journal of Medicine* 367 (2012): 1154–1158.

88. Frank Thompson, *Medicaid Politics: Federalism, Policy Durability, and Health Reform* (Washington, DC: Georgetown University Press, 2012); Alex Waddan, "Health Care Reform after the Supreme Court: Even More Known Unknowns," *Health, Economics, Politics, and Law* 8, no. 1 (2013): 139–143.

89. *National Federation of Independent Business et al. v. Sebelius et al.* 567 U.S. ___ (2012), 132 S.Ct.2566, http://www.supremecourt.gov/opinions/11pdf/11-393c3a2.pdf.

90. James Morone, "Seven Consequences of the Health Care Ruling," *New York Times*, June 28, 2012, accessed October 29, 2014, http://campaignstops.blogs.nytimes.com/2012/06/28/seven -consequences-of-the-health-care-ruling/.

91. Manny Fernandez, "Perry Declares Texas' Rejection of Health Care Law 'Intrusions,'" *New York Times*, July 9, 2010, A10.

92. Grace-Marie Turner, "*Hobby Lobby* Reminds Obama He Can't Just Interpret the Law How He Likes," *National Review Online*, June 30, 2014, accessed November 14, 2014, http://www .nationalreview.com/corner/381572/hobby-lobby-reminds-obama-he-cant-just-interpret-law -how-he-likes-grace-marie-turner.

93. Ibid.

94. Timothy Jost, "Subsidies and the Survival of the ACA: Divided Decisions on Premium

Tax Credits," *New England Journal of Medicine*, July 30, 2014, accessed November 2, 2014, http://www.nejm.org/doi/full/10.1056/NEJMp1408958.

95. *Halbig v. Burwell*, 14-5018 (D.C. Cir. 2014), 14–22.

96. *King v. Burwell*, 14-114, (4th Cir. 2014).

97. Adam Liptak, "Supreme Court Allows Nationwide Health Care Subsidies," *New York Times*, June 25, 2015, accessed July 1, 2015, http://www.nytimes.com/2015/06/26/us/obamacare-supreme-court.html.

98. Sandhya Somashekhar and Amy Goldstein, "Federal Appeals Courts Issue Contradictory Rulings on Health-Law Subsidies," *Washington Post*, July 22, 2014, accessed October 29, 2014, http://www.washingtonpost.com/national/health-science/federal-appeals-court-panel-deals-major-blow-to-health-law/2014/07/22/c86dd2ce-06a5-11e4-bbf1-cc51275e7f8f_story.html?wpisrc=nl%5fwonk.

99. Joseph White, "Muddling through the Muddled Middle," *Journal of Health Politics, Policy, and Law* 36, no. 3 (2011): 447. For a critique of the legislative process from the Left, see Matt Taibbi, "Sick and Wrong: How Washington Is Screwing Up Health Care Reform—and Why It May Take a Revolt to Fix It," *Rolling Stone*, September 3, 2009, accessed November 14, 2014, http://www.rollingstone.com/politics/news/sick-and-wrong-20100405.

3. HEALTH INSURANCE EXCHANGES

1. Ashley Lopez, "Gov. Rick Scott Takes Obamacare Navigators Fight to Congress," Florida Center for Investigative Journalism, last modified September 19, 2013, accessed June 7, 2014, http://fcir.org/2013/09/19/rick-scott-obamacare-navigators-congress/.

2. US Department of Health and Human Services, "A One-Page Guide to the Health Insurance Marketplace," accessed June 26, 2014, https://www.healthcare.gov/get-covered-a-1-page-guide-to-the-health-insurance-marketplace/.

3. William P. Brandon and Keith Carnes, "Federal Health Insurance Reform and 'Exchanges': Recent History," *Journal of Health Care for the Poor and Underserved* 25, no. 1 (2014): xxxvii.

4. Ibid., xlvi.

5. Sarah Dash, Kevin W. Lucia, Katie Keith, and Christine Monahan, *Implementing the Affordable Care Act: Key Design Decisions for State-based Exchanges* (New York: Commonwealth Fund, 2013).

6. Brandon and Carnes, "Federal Health Insurance Reform and 'Exchanges,'" xlvi.

7. Patient Protection and Affordable Care Act, Public Law 111-148, sec. 1501.

8. Alex Wayne, "Extra Obamacare Sign-Up Time Mulled to Help Taxpayers Avoid Fine," *Bloomberg*, February 13, 2015, accessed March 9, 2015, http://www.bloomberg.com/news/articles/2015-02-13/extra-obamacare-sign-up-time-mulled-to-help-taxpayers-avoid-fine.

9. Ibid., sec. 1301–1302.

10. Ibid., sec. 1303.

11. Ibid., sec. 1303, 1311, 1312, 1313, 1321, 1322, and 1323.

12. On credit claiming and blame avoidance, see R. Kent Weaver, "The Politics of Blame Avoidance," *Journal of Public Policy* 6, no. 4 (1986): 371–398.

13. David K. Jones, Katherine W. V. Bradley, and Jonathan Oberlander, "Pascal's Wager: Health-Insurance Exchanges, Obamacare, and the Republican Dilemma," *Journal of Health Poli-*

NOTES TO PAGES 64–68

tics, Policy, and Law 39, no. 1 (2014): 100; see also Alain C. Enthoven, "The History and Principles of Managed Competition," *Health Affairs* 12, Supplement 1 (1993): 24–48.

14. Jacob S. Hacker, *The Road to Nowhere: The Genesis of President Clinton's Plan for Health Security* (Princeton, NJ: Princeton University Press, 1996).

15. Brandon and Carnes, "Federal Health Insurance Reform and 'Exchanges,'" xxxvii.

16. Jones, Bradley, and Oberlander, "Pascal's Wager," 101; Jonathan Oberlander, "Long Time Coming: Why Health Care Reform Finally Passed," *Health Affairs* 29 (2010): 1112–1116.

17. Brandon and Carnes, "Federal Health Insurance Reform and 'Exchanges,'" liv.

18. Jones, Bradley, and Oberlander, "Pascal's Wager," 127.

19. John Dinan, "Implementing Health Reform: Intergovernmental Bargaining and the Affordable Care Act," *Publius: The Journal of Federalism* 44, no. 3 (2014): 401.

20. Dinan, "Implementing Health Reform"; see also John Dinan, "Shaping Health Reform: State Government Influence in the Patient Protection and Affordable Care Act," *Publius: The Journal of Federalism* 41, no. 3 (2011): 395–420.

21. Patient Protection and Affordable Care Act, sec. 1321.

22. *Halbig v. Burwell*, 758 F.3d 390 (D.C. Cir. 2014); *King v. Burwell*, 759 F.3d 358 (4th Cir. 2014).

23. See, for example, Rose Vaughn Williams to Timothy Geithner, Re: REG-131491-10 Public Hearing on Proposed Rulemaking for the Health Insurance Program Tax Credit, November 10, 2011; Michael Gargano to Kathleen Sebelius, letter, October 31, 2011; Georgia Health Insurance Exchange Advisory Committee, *Report to the Governor* 13, December 15, 2011; Nikki R. Haley to Jim DeMint, letter, July 2, 2012; South Carolina Health Planning Commission, *Improving the Healthcare Marketplace in South Carolina*, November 2011, http://doi.sc.gov/DocumentCenter/View/2534.

24. Joanne Young, "Heinemen Opts for Federal Health Care Exchange," *Lincoln Journal Star*, November 15, 2012, accessed January 19, 2015, http://journalstar.com/news/state-and-regional/statehouse/heineman-opts-for-federal-health-care-exchange/article_c8b80018-c57b-52c7-807c-807535e3533a.html.

25. *Oklahoma ex rel. Pruitt v. Burwell*, No. 6:11-cv-00030-RAW (E.D. Oklahoma September 19, 2012) (ECF No. 35); Governor Mary Fallin, "Governor Fallin Announces Extension of Insure Oklahoma," press release, September 6, 2013.

26. Dinan, "Implementing Health Reform."

27. Ibid., 5; see also Jones, Bradley, and Oberlander, "Pascal's Wager," 123.

28. On federal flexibility, see Simon Haeder and David Weimer, "You Can't Make Me Do It: State Implementation of Insurance Exchanges under the Affordable Care Act," *Public Administration Review* 73, no. S1 (2013): S34–S47.

29. Elizabeth Rigby and Jake Haselswerdt, "Hybrid Federalism, Partisan Politics, and Early Implementation of State Health Insurance Exchanges," *Publius: The Journal of Federalism* 43, no. 3 (2013): 387–388.

30. Ibid.

31. Dinan, "Implementing Health Reform."

32. Pear, cited in ibid., 6.

33. In April 2013, 52 percent of Californians supported the ACA, and 38 percent of them opposed it; these numbers remained relatively stable. Field Poll, *California Voter Views of the Affordable Care Act and Its Implementation* (Woodland Hills: California Wellness Foundation, 2013).

34. Jones, Bradley, and Oberlander, "Pascal's Wager," 111; Christina Jewett, "Schwarzenegger Approves New Health Exchanges, but Not without a Fight," *California Watch*, last modified

October 4, 2010, accessed June 7, 2014, http://californiawatch.org/dailyreport/schwarzenegger
-approves-new-health-exchanges-not-without-fight-5273.

35. Christina Jewett, "As Insurers Fight Back, Lawmakers Craft Agency to Manage Coverage,"
California Watch, last modified August 9, 2010, accessed June 7, 2014, http://californiawatch.org
/dailyreport/insurers-fight-back-lawmakers-craft-agency-manage-coverage-3738.

36. Teresa Casazza, Allan Zaremberg, and John Kabateck, "Open Letter to Governor Arnold
Schwarzenegger: Let's Get Health Care Reform Right," September 28, 2010, accessed June 7, 2014,
http://www.flashreport.org/files/2010093009300442.pdf.

37. Jones, Bradley, and Oberlander, "Pascal's Wager," 111.

38. Peter Long and Jonathan Gruber, "Projecting the Impact of the Affordable Care Act on
California," *Health Affairs* 30, no. 1 (2010): 63–70.

39. Andrew B. Bindman and Andreas G. Schneider, "Catching a Wave: Implementing Health
Care Reform in California," *New England Journal of Medicine* 364 (April 2011): 1487–1489.

40. David Gorn, "Exchange Picks New Name: Covered California," *CaliforniaHealthline,* last
modified November 1, 2012, accessed June 7, 2014, http://www.californiahealthline.org/capitol
-desk/2012/11/new-name-for-exchange-covered-california.

41. California State Auditor, "New High-Risk Entity: Covered California Appears Ready to
Operate California's First Statewide Health Insurance Exchange, but Critical Work and Some
Concerns Remain. Report 2013-602," July 18, 2013, accessed June 7, 2014, https://www.bsa.ca.gov
/pdfs/reports/2013-602.pdf.

42. Richard Scheffler and Jessica Foster, "Covered California: A Progress Report," last modified
February 2, 2014, accessed June 7, 2014, http://petris.org/wp-content/uploads/2014/02/Covered
-CA-Report-2-1-/www.bloomberg.com/news/2014–rts/2013-602.pdf -4-14_Final.pdf.

43. Tracy Seipel, "Obamacare Sign-ups Beat Projections in U.S., California," *San Jose Mercury
News,* April 17, 2014, accessed June 7, 2014, http://www.mercurynews.com/health/ci_25586338
/obamacare-california-sign-ups-exceed-3-million-private.

44. Ibid.

45. Association for Community Affiliated Plans, "ACAP Panels and Presentations," last modified August 30, 2010, accessed June 7, 2014, http://www.communityplans.net/NewsEvents/ACAP
PresentationsandPanels/tabid/368/Default.aspx.

46. For example, Affordable Insurance Exchanges: State Exchange Grantee, meeting of the
Center for Consumer Information and Insurance Oversight, September 19–20, 2011, accessed
June 7, 2014, http://www.cms.gov/CCIIO/Resources/Presentations/hie-fall-2011-grantee-meeting
.html; Affordable Insurance Exchanges: System-Wide Exchange, meeting of the Center for Consumer Information and Insurance Oversight, May 21–23, 2012, accessed June 7, 2014, http://www
.cms.gov/CCIIO/Resources/Presentations/hie-spring-2012-conference.html.

47. Arkansas Insurance Department, "Notes from CCIIO Meeting," Denver, Colorado, May
4–5, 2011, accessed June 7, 2014, http://hbe.arkansas.gov/denver.pdf. On Wisconsin, see Kaiser
Family Foundation, "State Exchange Profiles: Wisconsin," last modified December 11, 2012, accessed June 7, 2014, http://kff.org/health-reform/state-profile/state-exchange-profiles-wisconsin/.

48. Robert Pear and Reed Abelson, "Law Will Proceed, Administration Says," *New York
Times,* December 13, 2010, accessed June 7, 2014, http://www.nytimes.com/2010/12/14/health
/policy/14impact.html.

49. Ibid.

50. Jones, Bradley, and Oberlander, "Pascal's Wager," 106.

51. Webb Millsaps, "NAIC Approves 'Model Act' for State Insurance Exchanges," Health Care
Law Reform, last modified December 21, 2010, accessed June 7, 2014, http://www.healthcarelaw

reform.com/2010/12/articles/payorsmanaged-care/naic-approves-model-act-for-state-insurance
-exchanges/.

52. Ibid.

53. National Association of Insurance Commissioners to Donald Berwick, letter, October 5, 2011, accessed June 7, 2014, http://www.naic.org/documents/index_health_reform_111005_naic
_letter_centers_medicare_medicaid_services2.pdf.

54. Kaiser Family Foundation, "State Exchange Profiles: Kansas," last modified March 21, 2013, accessed June 7, 2014, http://kff.org/health-reform/state-profile/state-exchange-profiles-kansas/.

55. Kansas Insurance Department, "Comment on the Notice of Proposed Rulemaking by the Department of Health and Human Services (HHS), 45 CFR Parts 155 and 156 (CMS-9989-P) Patient Protection and Affordable Care Act; Establishment of Exchanges and Quali-fied Health Plans," last modified October 30, 2011, accessed June 7, 2014, http://www.regulations
.gov/#!documentDetail;D=HHS-OS-2011-0020-0461.

56. Kaiser Family Foundation, "State Exchange Profiles: Tennessee," last modified December 10, 2012, accessed June 7, 2014, http://kff.org/health-reform/state-profile/state-exchange-profiles
-tennessee/.

57. Department of Finance and Administration, Division of Health Care Finance and Admin-istration, *State of Tennessee's Comments on Proposed Rules for Exchanges and QHPs,* last modified October 31, 2011, accessed June 7, 2014, http://www.regulations.gov/#!documentDetail;D=HHS
-OS-2011-0020-2087.

58. Haeder and Weimer, "You Can't Make Me Do It," S43.

59. Rigby and Haselswerdt. "Hybrid Federalism, Partisan Politics, and Early Implementation of State Health Insurance Exchanges."

60. J. Lester Feder, "HHS May Have to Get 'Creative' on Exchange," *Politico,* August 16, 2011, ac-cessed October 24, 2014, http://www.politico.com/news/stories/0811/61513.html#ixzz3DJQJbtiS.

61. Annie L. Mach and C. Stephen Redhead, "Federal Funding for Health Insurance Ex-changes," Congressional Research Service, last modified July 28, 2014, accessed September 14, 2014, http://fas.org/sgp/crs/misc/R43066.pdf.

62. Emily Wagster Pettus, "Mississippi Can Try for Fed-State Health Exchange," *North-east Mississippi News,* February 11, 2013, accessed October 24, 2014, http://djournal.com/view
/full_story/21676156/article-Mississippi-can-try-for-fed-state-health-exchange?instance=home
_news_right.

63. Ibid.

64. Patient Protection and Affordable Care Act, sec. 1311(a), (b).

65. "AG Jim Hood Says Insurance Commissioner Mike Chaney Can Set Up Health Ex-change," *Mississippi Press,* January 15, 2013.

66. Phil Galewitz, "Cracks Appearing in GOP Opposition to Health Law," *Kaiser Health News,* last modified January 23, 2013, accessed October 24, 2014, http://www.kaiserhealthnews.org
/stories/2013/january/23/mississippi-exchange-gop-opposition-fading.aspx.

67. "Bryant-Chaney Dispute Has Insurance Exchange Plan Up in the Air," *Mississippi Busi-ness Journal,* January 4, 2013, accessed October 24, 2014, http://msbusiness.com/blog/2013/01/04
/bryant-chaney-dispute-has-insurance-exchange-plan-up-in-air/.

68. National Conference of State Legislatures, "State Legislation and Actions Opting Out or Opposing Certain Health Reforms," last modified July 2013, accessed June 7, 2014, http://www
.ncsl.org/documents/summit/summit2013/online-resources/state-legislation-opt-out.pdf.

69. National Conference of State Legislatures, "State Laws and Actions Challenging PPACA,"

last modified October 2014, accessed October 23, 2014, http://www.ncsl.org/research/health /state-laws-and-actions-challenging-ppaca.aspx.

70. Mary Agnes Carey, "HHS Seeking $1.5B in Funding to Run Federal Health Insurance Exchanges," *Kaiser Health News,* last modified April 11, 2013, accessed June 7, 2014, http://www .kaiserhealthnews.org/stories/2013/april/10/obama-budget-insurance-exchanges.aspx.

71. Amy Goldstein and Juliet Eilperin, "HealthCare.gov: How Political Fear Was Pitted against Technical Needs," *Washington Post,* November 2, 2013, accessed June 7, 2014, http:// www.washingtonpost.com/politics/challenges-have-dogged-obamas-health-plan-since-2010 /2013/11/02/453fba42-426b-11e3-a624-41d661b0bb78_story.html.

72. Feder, "HHS May Have to Get 'Creative' on Exchange."

73. Lori Montgomery and Philip Rucker, "House Passes GOP Spending Plan That Defunds Obamacare," *Washington Post,* September 20, 2013, accessed June 26, 2014, http://www .washingtonpost.com/politics/house-passes-gop-spending-plan-that-defunds-obamacare /2013/09/20/4019117c-21fe-11e3-b73c-aab60bf735d0_story.html.

74. Ibid.

75. Sarah Kliff, "Meet the Bureaucrats Now Deciding Obamacare's Fate," *Wonkblog,* November 18, 2013, accessed June 7, 2014, http://washingtonpost.com/blogs/wonkblog/wp/2013/11/18 /meet-the-bureaucrats-now-deciding-obamacares-fate/.

76. Elise Viebeck, "HHS Announces $1.5B for State Exchanges," *The Hill,* January 17, 2013, accessed June 7, 2014, http://thehill.com/policy/healthcare/277757-hhs-announces-15b-for-state -exchanges.

77. "Editorial: Scott's Campaign to Sabotage the Affordable Care Act," *Tampa Bay Times,* September 12, 2013.

78. "Stakeholder Conference on Exchanges," meeting of the Center for Consumer Information and Insurance Oversight, accessed June 7, 2014, http://cciio.cms.gov/resources/other /exchanges_video_8-30-2010.html.

79. Kaiser Family Foundation, "Essential Health Benefits: What Have States Decided for Their Benchmark?" last modified December 7, 2012, accessed June 7, 2014, http://kff.org/health-reform /fact-sheet/quick-take-essential-health-benefits-what-have-states-decided-for-their-bench mark/.

80. Philip Rocco, "Making Federalism Work? The Politics of Intergovernmental Collaboration and the PPACA," *Journal of Health and Human Services Administration,* 37 no. 4 (Spring 2015): 412–461.

81. Quoted in ibid.

82. American Legislative Exchange Council, "History," accessed June 7, 2014, http://www.alec .org/about-alec/history/.

83. American Legislative Exchange Council, *State Legislators Guide to Repealing ObamaCare,* accessed June 7, 2014, http://www.alec.org/wp-content/uploads/State_Leg_Guide_to_Repealing _ObamaCare.pdf.

84. American Legislative Exchange Council, "Health Care Freedom Act," accessed June 7, 2014, http://www.alec.org/model-legislation/health-care-freedom-act/.

85. Ed Pilkington, "Obamacare Faces New Threat at State Level from Corporate Interest Group ALEC," *Guardian,* November 20, 2013, accessed June 7, 2014, http://www.theguardian .com/world/2013/nov/20/obamacare-alec-republican-legislators.

86. Rigby and Haselswerdt, "Hybrid Federalism, Partisan Politics, and Early Implementation of State Health Insurance Exchanges," 378.

87. Ibid., 382.

88. Christie, quoted in ibid., 384.

89. Jackie Farwell, "LePage Won't Lift a Finger to Set Up Maine's Health Insurance Exchange," *Bangor Daily News*, November 15, 2012, accessed June 7, 2014, http://bangordailynews.com/2012 /11/15/health/lepage-wont-lift-a-finger-to-set-up-maines-health-insurance-exchange/.

90. Anna M. Tinsley, "Texas Light Bulb Bill Would Skirt Federal Plan," *McClatchy DC*, June 13, 2011, accessed October 24, 2014, http://www.mcclatchydc.com/2011/06/13/115661/texas-light -bulb-bill-would-skirt.html.

91. Emily Ramshaw, "Health Law Response Goes 2 Ways," *New York Times*, January 29, 2011, accessed June 7, 2014, http://www.nytimes.com/2011/01/30/us/30ttreform.html?_r=0.

92. "Perry Wrestles with His Own Healthcare Approach," *CBC DFW*, August 22, 2011, accessed June 7, 2014, http://dfw.cbslocal.com/2011/08/22/perry-wrestles-with-his-own-healthcare -approach/.

93. Office of Governor Rick Perry, "Gov. Perry: Texas Will Not Expand Medicaid or Implement Health Benefit Exchange," last modified July 9, 2012, accessed July 1, 2015, http://www.lrl .state.tx.us/scanned/govdocs/Rick%20Perry/2012/pressletter070912.pdf.

94. Christy Hoppe, "Poll: Texans Still Shun Obamacare, Worry about Jobs and Education," *Dallasnews.com*, October 1, 2013, accessed June 7, 2014, http://trailblazersblog.dallasnews .com/2013/10/texans-still-shun-obamacare-worry-about-jobs-and-education.html/.

95. Louise Norris, "Texas Exchange Has Largest Enrollment Spike in the Country during March and April," *Healthinsurance.org*, last modified May 4, 2013, accessed June 7, 2014, http:// www.healthinsurance.org/texas-state-health-insurance-exchange/.

96. Jay Hancock, "Blue Cross Blue Shield Bets Big on Obamacare Exchanges," *Kaiser Health News*, last modified June 21, 2013, accessed June 7, 2014, http://www.kaiserhealthnews.org/stories /2013/june/21/obama-administration-blue-cross-blue-shield-insurance-exchanges-market places.aspx.

97. Ibid.

98. David Maly, "Texas Prepares to Shutter High-Risk Insurance Pool," *Texas Tribune*, October 17, 2013, accessed June 7, 2014, http://www.texastribune.org/2013/10/17/texas-prepares -shutter-high-risk-insurance-pool/.

99. Vivian Ho, Elena Marks, and Patricia Gail Bray, "Issue Brief 3: Early Effects of the Affordable Care Act on Health Insurance Coverage in Texas for 2014 (Health Reform Monitoring Survey—Texas)," Baker Institute, accessed June 7, 2014, http://bakerinstitute.org/media/files /Research/f5635d5c/EHF_Issue_Brief_3new.pdf.

100. Jonathan Oberlander and Krista Perreira, "Implementing Obamacare in a Red State: Dispatch from North Carolina," *New England Journal of Medicine* 369, no. 26 (2013): 2469.

101. Ibid., 2469–2470.

102. Ibid., 2470.

103. Jones, Bradley, and Oberlander, "Pascal's Wager," 106.

104. Mark Binker, Matthew Burns, and Renee Chou, "McCrory Backs Bill to Stop Medicaid Expansion," *WRAL.com*, February 12, 2013, accessed June 7, 2014, http://www.wral.com/mccrory -backs-bill-to-stop-medicaid-expansion/12095491/.

105. Ibid.

106. Brandon and Carnes, "Federal Health Insurance Reform and 'Exchanges,'" lii.

107. Oberlander and Perreira, "Implementing Obamacare in a Red State," 2470.

108. Jason deBruyn, "N.C. Hit 145% of Its Obama's ACA Enrollment Goal," *Triangle Business Journal*, May 2, 2014, accessed June 7, 2014, http://www.bizjournals.com/triangle/blog/2014/05/n

-c-hit-145-of-its-obamas-aca-enrollmentgoal.html?page=all. Also see Linda J. Blumberg, John Holahan, Genevieve M. Kenney, Matthew Buettgens, Nathaniel Anderson, Hannah Recht, and Stephen Zuckerman, "Measuring Marketplace Enrollment Relative to Enrollment Projections: Update," Urban Institute, May 1, 2014, accessed June 7, 2014, http://www.urban.org/UploadedPDF/413112-Measuring-Marketplace-Enrollment-Relative-to-Enrollment-Projections-Update.pdf.

109. Sabrina Tavernise and Allison Kopicki, "Southerners Don't Like Obamacare. They Also Don't Want to Repeal It," *New York Times*, April 23, 2014.

110. Ibid.

111. Rigby and Haselswerdt, "Hybrid Federalism, Partisan Politics, and Early Implementation of State Health Insurance Exchanges," 384.

112. David Ramsey, "Arkansas Republicans Still Fighting Obamacare: Why Federal-Government-Hating State Republicans, with Direction from National Conservatives, Oppose the State-Run Exchange," *Arkansas Times*, December 26, 2012, accessed June 7, 2014, http://www.arktimes.com/arkansas/arkansas-republicans-still-fighting-obamacare/Content?oid=2588150.

113. Max Brantley, "The Feds Will Run Arkansas Insurance Exchanges," *Arkansas Times*, December 2, 2011, accessed June 7, 2014, http://www.arktimes.com/ArkansasBlog/archives/2011/12/02/the-feds-will-run-arkansas-insurance-exchanges.

114. Max Brantley, "Is a Health Exchange Back on for Arkansas?" *Arkansas Times*, November 16, 2012, accessed June 7, 2014, http://www.arktimes.com/ArkansasBlog/archives/2012/11/16/is-a-health-exchange-back-on-for-arkansas.

115. Mike Beebe to Kathleen Sebelius, letter, November 15, 2012, accessed June 7, 2014, http://posting.arktimes.com/images/blogimages/2012/11/16/1353092270-beebeletter.pdf.

116. Andrew DeMillo, "Beebe: Arkansas to Stick with Partnership Exchange," *Insurance Journal*, December 14, 2012, accessed July 1, 2015, http://www.insurancejournal.com/news/southcentral/2012/12/14/274136.htm.

117. Beebe to Sebelius.

118. Max Brantley, "Arkansas Cleared for Health Insurance Exchange; RAND Study Touts Benefits of Health Law in Arkansas," *Arkansas Times*, January 3, 2013, accessed June 7, 2014, http://www.arktimes.com/ArkansasBlog/archives/2013/01/03/arkansas-cleared-for-health-insurance-exchange.

119. Nic Horton, "John Burris: Against the Obamacare Exchange before He Was for It," Arkansas Project, last modified May 6, 2014, accessed June 7, 2014, http://www.thearkansasproject.com/john-burris-against-the-health-care-exchange-before-he-was-for-it/.

120. Kaiser Family Foundation, "State Exchange Profiles: Arkansas," last modified October 29, 2013, accessed June 7, 2014, http://kff.org/health-reform/state-profile/state-exchange-profiles-arkansas/.

121. Kaiser Family Foundation, "Marketplace Enrollment as a Share of the Potential Marketplace Population," last modified April 19, 2014, accessed June 7, 2014, http://kff.org/health-reform/state-indicator/marketplace-enrollment-as-a-share-of-the-potential-marketplace-population/.

122. David Weigel, "Swung State: For the First Time, Democrats Aren't Trying to Win Missouri's Electoral Votes. Why?" *Slate*, October 3, 2012, accessed June 7, 2014, http://www.slate.com/articles/news_and_politics/politics/2012/10/missouri_politics_why_the_swing_state_is_now_a_red_state_.html.

123. Elizabeth Crisp, "Poll Suggests Missourians Favor Medicaid Expansion," *St. Louis Post Dispatch*, December 11, 2012, accessed June 7, 2014, http://www.stltoday.com/news/local/govt-and-politics/elizabeth-crisp/poll-suggests-missourians-favor-medicaid-expansion/article_1fac4963-b312-575e-a47e-49e2158f259d.html.

124. Jessica Machetta, "Missourians Approve Prop C, the Health Care Freedom Act," *Missourinet.com*, last modified August 3, 2010, accessed June 7, 2014, http://www.missourinet.com /2010/08/03/missourians-approve-prop-c-the-health-care-freedom-act/.

125. Kaiser Family Foundation, "State Exchange Profiles: Missouri," last modified December 13, 2012, accessed June 7, 2014, http://kff.org/health-reform/state-profile/state-exchange-profiles -missouri/.

126. Ibid.

127. Wes Duplantier, "Proposition E Puts Health Care Back on Missouri Ballots," *Stlouis .cbslocal.com*, September 28, 2012, accessed June 7, 2014, http://stlouis.cbslocal.com/2012/09/28 /proposition-e-puts-health-care-back-on-missouri-ballots/.

128. "Missouri Health Exchange Referendum: 2012 Ballot Proposition E," *Focus St. Louis*, accessed June 7, 2014, http://www.focus-stl.org/?page=MOHealthExchange.

129. Missouri Foundation for Health, "Proposition E Summary: Health Insurance Exchange in Missouri—November 6, 2012," accessed June 7, 2014, http://www.mffh.org/mm/files/PropE Analysis.pdf.

130. Ibid.

131. Duplantier, "Proposition E Puts Health Care Back on Missouri Ballots."

132. Susan Talve, president of Missouri Health Care for All, quoted in ibid.

133. Quoted in ibid.

134. Virginia Young, "Missouri Consumers in the Dark as Health Insurance Exchange Nears," *St. Louis Post Dispatch*, August 14, 2013, accessed June 7, 2014, http://www.stltoday.com/news /local/govt-and-politics/political-fix/missouri-consumers-in-the-dark-as-health-insurance -exchange-nears/article_d3d1adcf-6aa9-5503-b114-dc7b00648ea8.html.

135. Elizabeth Crisp, "Gov. Jay Nixon Notifies Feds That Missouri Won't Create Insurance Exchange," *St. Louis Post Dispatch*, November 16, 2012, accessed June 7, 2014, http://www.stltoday .com/news/local/govt-and-politics/political-fix/gov-jay-nixon-notifies-feds-that-missouri-won -t-create/article_2d6815a2-f5ef-588f-9cbb-3189da9763f2.html.

136. Jay Nixon to Kathleen Sebelius, letter, November 16, 2012, accessed June 7, 2014, http:// www.stltoday.com/online/media/gov-nixon-s-letter-on-the-insurance-exchange/pdf_7422cfd5 -6f0c-5ee9-9adf-d65c19ce4c53.html.

137. Robert Pear, "Missouri Citizens Face Obstacles to Coverage," *New York Times*, August 2, 2013, accessed June 7, 2014, http://www.nytimes.com/2013/08/03/us/missouri-citizens-face -obstacles-to-coverage.html?_r=1&.

138. Herb B. Kuhn, president of the Missouri Hospital Association, quoted in ibid.

139. Michael Boldin, "Missouri Bill Would Gut Obamacare," *Washington Times*, December 27, 2013, http://communities.washingtontimes.com/neighborhood/view-tenth/2013/dec/27 /missouri-bill-would-gut-obamacare/.

140. Alex Nussbaum and Andrew Zajac, "Law Restricting Obamacare Navigators Blocked by Missouri Judge," *Bloomberg.com*, January 24, 2013, accessed June 7, 2014, http://www.bloomberg .com/news/2014-01-23/missouri-law-restricting-obamacare-guides-blocked-by-judge-1.html.

141. Carla Anderson, "Missouri Health Plan Enrollment, Medicaid Qualifications Exceed 100,000," *Healthinsurance.org*, last modified April 24, 2014, accessed June 7, 2014, http://www .healthinsurance.org/missouri-state-health-insurance-exchange/.

4. MEDICAID EXPANSION

1. Shanna Rose, *Financing Medicaid: Federalism and the Growth of America's Health Care Safety Net* (Ann Arbor: University of Michigan Press, 2013), 11.

2. Laura Katz Olson, *The Politics of Medicaid* (New York: Columbia University Press, 2010), 223.

3. Kaiser Commission on Medicaid and the Uninsured, *Medicaid: A Primer*, March 2013, accessed November 14, 2014, http://kaiserfamilyfoundation.files.wordpress.com/2010/06/7334-05 .pdf.

4. American Legislative Exchange Council, *The State Legislators' Guide to Repealing Obama-Care* (Washington, DC: ALEC, 2011), 2.

5. David Remnick, "Going the Distance: On and off the Road with Barack Obama," *New Yorker,* January 27, 2014, accessed November 14, 2014, http://www.newyorker.com/magazine /2014/01/27/going-the-distance-2?currentPage=all.

6. At the end of August 2014, Pennsylvania became the twenty-seventh state, along with the District of Columbia, to agree to participate in the expansion, reducing the number of nonparticipating states to twenty-three. At that point three states, Indiana, Michigan, and Utah, were actively considering expansion, and by June 2015 Indiana and Michigan had expanded their programs.

7. Renee Landers, "The Denouement of the Supreme Court's ACA Drama," *New England Journal of Medicine* 366, no. 3 (2012): 198–199; Alex Waddan, "Health Care after the Supreme Court: Even More Known Unknowns," *Health, Economics, Politics, and Law* 8, no. 1 (2013): 139–143.

8. Stan Dorn, Megan McGrath, and John Holahan, "What Is the Result of States Not Expanding Medicaid?" Robert Wood Johnson Foundation and the Urban Institute, August 2014, http:// www.urban.org/UploadedPDF/413192-What-Is-the-Result-of-States-Not-Expanding-Medicaid .pdf.

9. Lawrence Jacobs and Timothy Callaghan, "Why States Expand Medicaid: Party, Resource, and History," *Journal of Health Politics, Policy, and Law* 38, no. 5 (2013): 1040.

10. Michael Doonan, *American Federalism in Practice: The Formulation and Implementation of Contemporary Health Policy* (Washington, DC: Brookings Institution, 2013), 124. See also Sarah Kliff, "Republican Governors Have Found Something They Like about Obamacare," Vox.com, May 20, 2014, accessed November 14, 2014, http://www.vox.com/2014/5/20/5730798/republican -governors-have-found-something-they-like-about-obamacare.

11. Tom Daschle with David Nather, *Getting It Done: How Obama and Congress Finally Broke the Stalemate to Make Way for Health Care Reform* (New York: Thomas Dunne Books, 2010).

12. Sharon K. Long, "On the Road to Universal Coverage: Impacts of Reform in Massachusetts at One Year," *Health Affairs* 27, no. 4 (2008): 270–284.

13. Lawrence Brown and Michael Sparer, "Poor Program's Progress: The Unanticipated Politics of Medicaid Policy," *Health Affairs* 22, no. 1 (2003): 31–44. See also Colleen Grogan and Eric M. Patashnik, "Between Welfare Medicine and Mainstream Entitlement: Medicaid at the Crossroads," *Journal of Health Politics, Policy, and Law* 28, no. 5 (2003): 821–858.

14. Charles Kahn and Ronald Pollack, "Building a Consensus for Expanding Health Coverage," *Health Affairs* 20, no. 1 (2001): 40–48.

15. James Douglas and Joe Manchin III to Max Baucus and Charles Grassley, letter, July 20, 2009, accessed November 14, 2014, http://www.nga.org/cms/home/federal-relations/nga-letters /executive-committee-letters/co12-content/main-content-list/title_july-20-2009-1.html.

16. Rose, *Financing Medicaid*, 230–234.

17. Congressional Budget Office (CBO), "H.R. 4872, Reconciliation Act of 2010," March 18, 2010, http://www.cbo.gov/ftpdocs/113xx/doc11355/hr4872.pdf.

18. Kaiser Commission on Medicaid and the Uninsured, *Medicaid: A Primer*, 8.

19. Samantha Artiga and Robin Rudowitz, "Medicaid Enrollment under the Affordable Care Act: Understanding the Numbers," Kaiser Family Foundation, last modified January 29, 2014, ac-

cessed November 14, 2014, http://kff.org/health-reform/issue-brief/medicaid-enrollment-under -the-affordable-care-act-understanding-the-numbers/.

20. Frank Thompson, *Medicaid Politics: Federalism, Policy Durability, and Health Reform* (Washington, DC: Georgetown University Press, 2012), 92.

21. Kaiser Commission on Medicaid and the Uninsured, *Medicaid Eligibility, Enrollment Simplification, and Coordination under the Affordable Care Act: A Summary of CMS's March 23, 2012, Final Rule,* last modified December 2012, accessed November 14, 2014, http://kaiserfamily foundation.files.wordpress.com/2013/04/8391.pdf.

22. J. McDonough, "The Road Ahead for the Affordable Care Act," *New England Journal of Medicine* 367, no. 3 (2012): 199–210.

23. Kaiser Commission on Medicaid and the Uninsured, *Medicaid: An Overview of Spending on "Mandatory" vs. "Optional" Populations and Services,* last modified June 2005, accessed November 14, 2014, http://www.kaiserfamilyfoundation.files.wordpress.com/2013/01/medicaid -an-overview-of-spending-on.pdf.

24. Douglas Jaenicke and Alex Waddan, "Recent Incremental Health Care Reforms in the US: A Way Forward or False Promise?" *Policy and Politics* 34, no. 2 (2006): 241–263.

25. Thompson, *Medicaid Politics,* 60–62.

26. Michael Greve and Philip Wallach, *As Arizona Goes, So Goes the Nation: How Medicaid Ruins the States' Fiscal Health* (Washington, DC: American Enterprise Institute, 2008), 7, http:// www.aei.org/files/2008/07/17/20080717_0623308HPOJuly_g.pdf.

27. Amy Goldstein and Dan Balz, "Governors Differ on Extent of Flexibility for Medic- aid," *Washington Post,* February 27, 2011, accessed November 14, 2014, http://www.washington post.com/wp-dyn/content/article/2011/02/27/AR2011022703688.html?wpisrc=nl_politics; see also Peter Orszag, "How Health Care Can Save or Sink America," *Foreign Affairs* 90, no. 4 (2011): 42–56.

28. Charles Barrilleaux and Paul Brace, "Notes from the Laboratories of Democracy: State Government Enactments of Market- and State-Based Health Insurance Reforms in the 1990s," *Journal of Health Politics, Policy, and Law* 32, no. 4 (2007): 658.

29. National Association of State Budget Officers, "Summary: NASBO State Expenditures Report," last modified December 2010, accessed November 14, 2014, http://www.nasbo.org/Link Click.aspx?fileticket=HSlQhWvejXA%3d&tabid=38.

30. Robert Pear, "In Health Care Ruling, Vast Implications for Medicaid," *New York Times,* June 16, 2012, A12.

31. Kevin Sack, "For Governors, Medicaid Looks Ripe for Slashing," *New York Times,* January 29, 2011, A1.

32. Sandra Deckker, "In 2011 Nearly One-Third of Physicians Said They Would Not Accept New Medicaid Patients, but Rising Fees May Help," *Health Affairs* 31, no. 8 (2012): 1673–1679. Deckker's study found that 31 percent of doctors across the United States would not accept new Medicaid patients, though this varied hugely from state to state. It should be emphasized that there was not a correlation between the generosity of payments states made to doctors through Medicaid and the overall scale of a state Medicaid program.

33. Thomas Friedman, "President Allows States Flexibility on Medicaid Funds," *New York Times,* February 2, 1993, accessed November 14, 2014, http://www.nytimes.com/1993/02/02/us /president-allows-states-flexibility-on-medicaid-funds.html. Interestingly, internal Clinton White House documents reveal that the administration quickly began to worry that the waivers and flexibility it gave the states might undermine its effort at comprehensive national health care reform by encouraging governors to see reform as a state rather than federal matter. See Rose,

Financing Medicaid, 180. For a fuller discussion of the use of waivers in the Clinton era, see Rose, *Financing Medicaid,* 159–184.

34. Rose, *Financing Medicaid,* 164.

35. US Government Accountability Office (GAO), *Medicaid Demonstration Waivers: Lack of Opportunity for Public Input during Federal Approval Process Still a Concern,* July 24, 2007, accessed November 14, 2014, http://www.gao.gov/assets/100/95034.pdf.

36. On types of waiver authority available to place Medicaid enrollees into managed-care organizations, see Centers for Medicare and Medicaid Services, *Medicaid.gov, Managed Care,* accessed November 14, 2014, http://www.medicaid.gov/Medicaid-CHIP-Program-Information/By -Topics/Delivery-Systems/Managed-Care/Managed-Care.html.

37. Michael Sparer, "Federalism and the Patient Protection and Affordable Care Act of 2010: The Founding Fathers Would Not Be Surprised," *Journal of Health Policy, Politics, and Law* 36, no. 3 (2011): 462–468.

38. Jonathan Oberlander, "Health Reform Interrupted: The Unraveling of the Oregon Health Plan," *Health Affairs* 26, no. 1 (2007): 96–105.

39. *National Federation of Independent Business (NFIB) et al. v. Sebelius et al.,* 567 U.S. (2012), 132 S.Ct.2566, 53–54, http://www.supremecourt.gov/opinions/11pdf/11-393c3a2.pdf.

40. Landers, "The Denouement of the Supreme Court's ACA Drama," 2012.

41. *NFIB v. Sebelius,* 51.

42. Wendy Mariner, Leonard Glantz, and George Annas, "Reframing Federalism: The Affordable Care Act (and Broccoli) in the Supreme Court," *New England Journal of Medicine* 367, no. 12 (2012): 1156–1157. These authors added that the "Court had never before found a federal spending program to be coercive, and most scholars believed coercion to be an illusory standard that the Court would not apply."

43. *NFIB v. Sebelius,* 52.

44. Jonathan Martin, "Health Law Is Dividing Republican Governors," *New York Times,* November 22, 2013, A14.

45. Timothy Jost and Sara Rosenbaum, "The Supreme Court and the Future of Medicaid," *New England Journal of Medicine* 367, no. 11 (2012): 985.

46. Timothy Jost, "Implementing Health Reform: State Innovation and Medicaid Waivers," *Health Affairs Blog,* February 23, 2012, accessed November 14, 2014, http://healthaffairs.org /blog/2012/02/23/implementing-health-reform-state-innovation-and-medicaid-waivers/.

47. Dennis Andrulis, Nadia Siddiqui, Maria Cooper, and Lauren Jahnke, "Report No. 2: Supporting and Transitioning the Health Care Safety Net," Texas Health Institute, Affordable Care Act and Racial and Ethnic Health Equity Series, August 2013, accessed November 14, 2014, http:// www.texashealthinstitute.org/uploads/1/3/5/3/13535548/aca_safetynet_report-08_02_2013final .pdf.

48. Kaiser Family Foundation, Kaiser Health Tracking Poll, last modified March 2013, accessed November 14, 2014, http://kff.org/health-reform/poll-finding/march-2013-tracking-poll/.

49. Dennis Smith and Edmund Haislmaier, "Medicaid Meltdown: Dropping Medicaid Could Save States $1 Trillion," Heritage Foundation, last modified December 1, 2009, accessed November 14, 2014, http://www.heritage.org/research/reports/2009/11/medicaid-meltdown-dropping -medicaid-could-save-states-1-trillion.

50. Nevada Department of Health and Human Services and Division of Health Care Financing and Policy, *Medicaid Opt Out White Paper,* January 22, 2010, accessed November 14, 2014, http://media.lasvegassun.com/media/pdfs/blogs/documents/2010/01/28/medcaid0128.pdf.

51. Ibid., 19–23.

52. Robert Pear, "Republican Governor of Florida Says State Won't Expand Medicaid," *New York Times*, July 3, 2012, A10. In his blow-by-blow account of the introduction of the ACA, journalist Steven Brill confirmed that the White House did assume that states, "even those run by the most conservative Republicans," would expand their Medicaid programs. Brill, *America's Bitter Pill: Money, Politics, Backroom Deals, and the Fight to Fix Our Broken Healthcare System* (New York: Random House, 2015), 258.

53. Kathleen Sebelius to all US governors, letter, July 10, 2012, accessed November 14, 2014, http://www.ncsl.org/documents/health/SecSeb_Ltr_GOV.pdf.

54. Dorn, McGrath, and Holahan, "What Is the Result of States Not Expanding Medicaid?"

55. "Gov. Nikki Haley: We Will Not Expand Medicaid on President Obama's Watch," CBS Atlanta, March 30, 2013, accessed November 14, 2014, http://atlanta.cbslocal.com/2013/03/30/gov-nikki-haley-we-will-not-expand-medicaid-on-president-obamas-watch/.

56. Trip Gabriel, "Expansion of Medicaid Is Now Set for Ohioans," *New York Times*, October 22, 2013, A12.

57. "Gov. Kasich Explains Why He Expanded Medicaid in Ohio," Real Clear Politics, November 16, 2013, http://www.realclearpolitics.com/video/2013/11/16/gov_john_kasich_explains_why_he_expanded_medicaid_in_ohio.html.

58. Phil Galewitz, "Sebelius Signal to States: Don't Roll Back Medicaid Eligibility," *Kaiser Health News*, last modified July 11, 2012, accessed November 14, 2014, http://www.kaiserhealthnews.org/stories/2012/july/11/sebelius-letter-governors-health-law.aspx.

59. Peter Frost, "Quinn Signs Illinois Medicaid Expansion Bill," *Chicago Tribune*, July 22, 2013, accessed November 14, 2014, http://articles.chicagotribune.com/2013-07-22/business/chi-illinois-medicaid-expansion-20130722_1_medicaid-expansion-medicaid-coverage-lincoln-health.

60. Throughout the period in which the California government made plans for the full Medicaid expansion, there were a series of arguments about methods of cost containment in the state Medicaid program. For example, Governor Jerry Brown clashed with the Obama administration when the state requested permission to charge Medi-Cal beneficiaries copays for visits to the emergency room. Richard Simon, "Gov. Meets with Congressional Delegation, Still Hopeful on Medi-Cal," *Los Angeles Times*, February 27, 2012, accessed November 14, 2014, http://latimesblogs.latimes.com/california-politics/2012/02/jerry-brown-meets-with-delegationl-on-medi-cal.html. State officials made no pretense that their proposals were driven by consideration of the best interests of their Medicaid beneficiaries. California Medicaid director Toby Douglas lamented, "We are having to make proposals that are not the best choices for our most vulnerable beneficiaries," but "given our limited resources, they are the best choices for the State of California." Sack, "For Governors, Medicaid Looks Ripe for Slashing".

61. Stu Woo, "Schwarzenegger Airs Medicaid Cost Concerns, but Still Backs Action," *Wall Street Journal*, October 28, 2009, accessed November 14, 2014, http://online.wsj.com/news/articles/SB125666629178410871.

62. Jane Norman, "Schwarzenegger Protests Cost of Medicaid Expansion in Overhaul," Commonwealth Fund, last modified December 28, 2009, accessed November 14, 2014, http://www.commonwealthfund.org/publications/newsletters/washington-health-policy-in-review/2009/dec/december-28–2009/schwarzenegger-protests-cost-of-medicaid-expansion-in-overhaul.

63. Julian Pecquet, "Schwarzenegger Endorses Healthcare Law, Says California Will Move Ahead Responsibly," *The Hill*, April 29, 2010, accessed November 14, 2014, http://thehill.com/homenews/news/95221-schwarzenegger-endorses-healthcare-law-says-california-will-move-ahead-responsibly.

64. Ibid.

65. Peter Harbage and Meredith Ledford King, "A Bridge to Reform: California's Medicaid Section 1115 Waiver," California Healthcare Foundation, last modified October 2012, accessed November 14, 2014, http://www.chcf.org/publications/2012/10/bridge-to-reform.

66. State of California, *California Section 1115 Comprehensive Demonstration Project Waiver: A Bridge to Reform—A Section 1115 Waiver Proposal,* June 2010, accessed November 14, 2014, http://www.dhcs.ca.gov/provgovpart/Documents/A%20Bridge%20to%20Reform%206-10-2010.pdf.

67. Kaiser Commission on Medicaid and the Uninsured, *Key Facts on California's 'Bridge to Reform' Medicaid Demonstration Waiver,* October 2011, accessed November 14, 2014, http://kaiserfamilyfoundation.files.wordpress.com/2013/01/8197-fs.pdf.

68. Kaiser Family Foundation, *States Getting a Jump Start on Health Reform's Medicaid Expansion,* last modified April 2, 2012, accessed November 14, 2014, http://kff.org/health-reform/issue-brief/states-getting-a-jump-start-on-health/.

69. Sarah Kliff, "Obamacare's Medicaid Expansion Already Covering a Half-Million Americans," *Washington Post,* July 3, 2012, accessed November 14, 2014, http://www.washingtonpost.com/blogs/wonkblog/wp/2012/07/03/obamacares-medicaid-expansion-already-covering-a-half-million-americans/.

70. Michael Mishak, "Counties Express Concern about Medi-Cal Expansion," *Los Angeles Times,* January 29, 2013, http://latimesblogs.latimes.com/california-politics/2013/01/counties-express-concerns-about-medi-cal-expansion.html.

71. Patrick McGreevy, "Gov. Jerry Brown Calls for Special Session of Legislature on Healthcare," *Los Angeles Times,* January 24, 2013, accessed November 14, 2014, http://latimesblogs.latimes.com/california-politics/2013/01/jerry-brown-legislature-healthcare.html.

72. Autumn Kieber-Emmons, "Medicaid Expansion and Reform: Hopes and Lessons from California," *Health Affairs Blog,* July 14, 2011, accessed November 14, 2014, http://healthaffairs.org/blog/2011/07/14/medicaid-expansion-and-reform-hopes-and-lessons-from-california/.

73. Tina Hossain, "Medi-Cal Expansion: The Road Ahead, Los Angeles Area Chamber of Commerce," May 7, 2014, accessed November 14, 2014, http://www.lachamber.com/blog/detail/2014/05/07/health-care-waiting-room/medi-cal-expansion-the-road-ahead/.

74. Chris Megerian, "New Budget Expands Healthcare in California," *Los Angeles Times,* June 27, 2013, accessed November 14, 2014, http://www.latimes.com/local/lanow/la-me-pc-jerry-brown-california-budget-20130627-story.html.

75. David Siders, "Field Poll: Support Grows in California for Federal Health Law," *Sacramento Bee,* August 20, 2012, 3A.

76. Jason Millman and Kyle Cheney, "Jan Brewer Wins Medicaid Expansion in Arizona," *Politico,* June 13, 2013, accessed November 14, 2014, http://www.politico.com/story/2013/06/arizona-medicaid-expansion-jan-brewer-92723.html.

77. American Legislative Exchange Council, *The State Legislators Guide to Repealing Obama-Care* (Washington, DC: ALEC, 2011), 13.

78. Rose, *Financing Medicaid,* 162.

79. Northern Arizona Regional Behavioral Health Authority, Arizona Chamber Foundation, *Understanding AHCCCS and Proposition 204,* accessed November 14, 2014, http://www.narbha.org/includes/media/docs/Understanding-AHCCCS-and-Proposition-204.pdf.

80. Ibid.

81. Ibid.

82. For a review of the boom and bust of Arizona's economy and the state fiscal capacity, see Matthew Murray with Kristin Borns, Sue Clark-Johnson, Mark Muro, and Jennifer Vey, *Structur-*

ally Unbalanced: Cyclical and Structural Deficits in Arizona, Brookings Mountain West/Morrison Institute for Public Policy, January 2011, accessed November 14, 2014, http://www.brookings.edu/~/media/research/files/papers/2011/1/05%20state%20budgets/0105_state_budgets_arizona.pdf.

83. Greve and Wallach, *As Arizona Goes, So Goes the Nation,* 4.

84. Kevin Sack, "Arizona Drops Children's Health Program," *New York Times,* March 19, 2010, A17.

85. Thompson, *Medicaid Politics,* 191.

86. Kevin Sack, "Sebelius Clears the Way for Arizona to Shed Adults from Medicaid," *New York Times,* February 16, 2011, A17.

87. Editors, "Brewer's Price," *National Review Online,* January 16, 2013, accessed November 14, 2014, http://www.nationalreview.com/articles/337788/brewer-s-price-editors.

88. Christina Corieri, "Ten Reasons to Decline Medicaid Expansion in Arizona," Goldwater Institute, last modified March 22, 2013, accessed November 14, 2014, http://www.goldwaterinstitute.org/10-reasons-to-decline-medicaid-expansion.

89. Americans for Prosperity–Arizona, *Refutation of Gov. Brewer's Medicaid Expansion Arguments,* last modified January 16, 2013, accessed November 14, 2014, http://americansforprosperity.org/arizona/legislativealerts/refutation-of-gov-jan-brewers-medicaid-expansion-arguments/.

90. Janice K. Brewer, Office of the Arizona Governor, "Governor Brewer's Medicaid Plan: The Conservative Choice for America," accessed November 14, 2014, http://www.azgovernor.gov/Medicaid.asp.

91. Fernanda Santos, "G.O.P. in Arizona Is Pushed to Expand Medicaid," *New York Times,* March 11, 2013, A11. This claim by Betlach was somewhat misleading because the Arizona waiver under Proposition 204 covered people up to 100 percent of the FPL rather than the 138 percent in the ACA.

92. Ibid.

93. Mary K. Reinhart and Yvonne Wingett Sanchez, "Brewer Advisers Form Health Pact to Push to Expand Medicaid," *Republic,* August 12, 2012, accessed November 14, 2014, http://www.azcentral.com/news/politics/articles/20120810brewer-health-pact-formed.html.

94. Howard Fischer, "Brewer Working New Path to Expand Arizona Medicaid Program," *East Valley Tribune,* May 7, 2013, accessed November 14, 2014, http://m.eastvalleytribune.com/arizona/politics/article_10782280-b74d-11e2-a159-0019bb2963f4.html?mode=jqm.

95. National Council of State Legislatures (NCSL), *Statevote 2012,* accessed November 14, 2014, http://www.ncsl.org/research/elections-and-campaigns/statevote.aspx. The previous majorities had been forty to nineteen in the House (with one vacancy at the time of the election) and twenty-one to nine in the Senate.

96. Mary Reinhart, "Brewer Signs into Law Arizona's Medicaid Program," *Republic,* June 18, 2013, accessed November 14, 2014, http://www.azcentral.com/news/politics/articles/20130617brewer-signs-law-arizona-medicaid-program.html.

97. Fernanda Santos, "Republicans in Arizona Are at Odds on Medicaid," *New York Times,* July 22, 2013, A10. In fact, all the Republicans who voted for the expansion won their primary reelection contests in summer 2014.

98. Mary Reinhart, "Competing Medicaid Petitions Cause Confusion, Consternation," *Republic,* July 6, 2013, accessed November 14, 2014, http://www.azcentral.com/news/politics/articles/20130703arizona-medicaid-petitions-confusion.html.

99. Paige Lavender, "Jan Brewer Sued over Arizona Medicaid Law," *Huffington Post,* September 13, 2013, accessed November 14, 2014, http://www.huffingtonpost.com/2013/09/13/jan-brewer-sued_n_3921086.html.

100. Mitch Daniels, "An Obamacare Appeal from the States," *Wall Street Journal*, February 7, 2011, accessed November 14, 2014, http://online.wsj.com/news/articles/SB10001424052748703652 104576122172835584158?mg=reno64-.

101. Smith and Haislmaier, "Medicaid Meltdown."

102. American Legislative Exchange Council, *State Legislators Guide to Repealing Obama-Care*, 17.

103. Rose, *Financing Medicaid*, 243.

104. Republican Governors Association, "RGA Letter on Medicaid and Exchanges to President Obama," accessed November 14, 2014, http://www.rga.org/homepage/rga-letter-on-medicaid -and-exchanges-to-president-obama/.

105. Tony Pugh, "Despite Health Challenges, Southern States Resist Medicaid Expansion," *Miami Herald*, July 3, 2013, accessed November 14, 2014, http://www.miamiherald.com/incoming /article1950163.html.

106. American Legislative Exchange Council, *State Legislators Guide to Repealing Obama-Care*, 16.

107. American Legislative Exchange Council, *Resolution Opposing PPACA Medicaid Expansion*, last modified June 2013, accessed November 14, 2014, http://www.alec.org/model-legislation /resolution-opposing-ppaca-medicaid-expansion/.

108. Olson, *Politics of Medicaid*, 91.

109. Mario Moretto, "LePage Vetoes Medicaid Expansion, Calling the Effort 'Ruinous' for Maine's Future," *Bangor Daily News*, April 9, 2014, accessed November 14, 2014, http://bangordaily news.com/2014/04/09/politics/lepage-vetoes-medicaid-expansion-calling-the-effort-ruinous -for-maines-future/.

110. Martin, "Health Law Is Dividing Republican Governors."

111. Santos, "Republicans in Arizona Are at Odds on Medicaid."

112. Martin, "Health Law Is Dividing Republican Governors."

113. Jeffrey Young, "Dennis Daugaard, South Dakota Governor, Rejects Obamacare Medicaid Expansion," *Huffington Post*, December 5, 2012, accessed November 14, 2014, http://www.huffing tonpost.com/2012/12/05/dennis-daugaard-obamacare-rejects-medicaid_n_2244970.html.

114. Jay Root and Bobby Blanchard, "In Debate, Abbott Gets Aggressive, Davis Stays That Way," *Texas Tribune*, September 30, 2014, accessed November 14, 2014, http://www.texastribune .org/2014/09/30/abbott-gets-aggressive-davis-stays-way/.

115. Rick Perry, Office of the Governor, "Statement by Gov. Rick Perry on Passage of Federal Health Care Bill," March 21, 2010, accessed November 14, 2014, http://governor.state.tx.us/news /press-release/14396/.

116. Kevin Sack, "Texas Battles Health Law Even as It Follows It," *New York Times*, July 18, 2010, A10.

117. Emily Ramshaw, "Lawmakers Discussing Dropping Health Care Program," *Texas Tribune*, November 6, 2010, accessed November 14, 2014, http://www.texastribune.org/2010/11/06 /lawmakers-discussing-dropping-health-care-program/.

118. Texas Health and Human Services Commission, "Impact on Texas If Medicaid Is Eliminated," 2009, accessed November 14, 2014, https://www.hhsc.state.tx.us/HB-497_122010.pdf. The report was initially based on the idea of a change in federal policy but was amended to reflect the impact of a withdrawal initiated by the state. For a summary of its findings, see Anne Dunkelberg, "Let's Have an 'Adult Conversation' about Opting Out of Medicaid," last modified December 10, 2010, accessed November 14, 2014, http://ccf.georgetown.edu/ccf-resources/an_adult_conversa tion_about_opting_out_of_medicaid/.

119. Emily Ramshaw and Marilyn Werber Serafini, "State Keeps Pressing for Waiver to Change Medicaid, but Success Is Unlikely," *New York Times,* February 18, 2011, A25.

120. Kaiser Commission on Medicaid and the Uninsured, *Where Are States Today?* The coverage of parents of dependent children is a useful marker of state generosity because it is an area where states have considerable discretion. The raw numbers, however, should be treated with some caution because many states had some limited extra coverage in some circumstances. For example, in Louisiana, a specific section 1115 waiver meant that parents of dependent children in Greater New Orleans were eligible for some limited coverage with incomes up to 200 percent of the FPL.

121. Emily Ramshaw and Marilyn Werber Serafini, "States' Woes Spur Medicaid Drop Out Talk," *Kaiser Health News,* last modified November 12, 2010, accessed November 14, 2014, http://www.kaiserhealthnews.org/stories/2010/november/12/medicaid-drop-out.aspx.

122. Kaiser Family Foundation, "Health Insurance Coverage of the Total Population, 2013," accessed November 14, 2014, http://kff.org/other/state-indicator/total-population/.

123. Dorn, McGrath, and Holahan, "What Is the Result of States Not Expanding Medicaid?"

124. Rick Perry to Kathleen Sebelius, letter, July 9, 2012, accessed November 14, 2014, http://governor.state.tx.us/files/press-office/0-sebeliuskathleen201207090024.pdf.

125. Becca Aaronson, "Democrats Expect a Deal on Medicaid Despite Perry," *New York Times,* December 2, 2012, A39.

126. Ross Ramsey, "UT/TT Poll: Texans Like Parts of Federal Health Law," *Texas Tribune,* November 6, 2013, accessed November 14, 2014, http://www.texastribune.org/2013/11/06/uttt-poll -texans-parts-federal-health-law/.

127. David Mildenberg, "Perry Pressured by Texas Businesses over Medicaid Refusal," *Bloomberg,* March 19, 2013, accessed November 14, 2014, http://www.bloomberg.com/news/2013-03-19 /perry-pressured-by-texas-businesses-over-medicaid-refusal.html.

128. Ramsey, "UT/TT Poll."

129. Kelly Kennedy, "Medicaid Expansion Gap Could Leave Poor Shortchanged," *USA Today,* September 5, 2013, accessed November 14, 2014, http://www.usatoday.com/story/news /politics/2013/09/05/100-percent-medicaid/2749143/.

130. Thompson, *Medicaid Politics,* 194.

131. David Weigel, "The Hardest Sell," Slate.com, August 24, 2010, http://www.slate.com /articles/news_and_politics/politics/2010/08/the_hardest_sell.html.

132. Kevin Sack, David Herszenhorn, and Robert Pear, "States Diverge on How to Deal with Health Care Ruling," *New York Times,* February 2, 2011, A16.

133. Robert Pear, "Republican Governor of Florida Says State Won't Expand Medicaid," *New York Times,* July 3, 2012, A10.

134. Lizette Alvarez, "In Reversal, Florida Says It Will Expand Medicaid," *New York Times,* February 21, 2010, A13.

135. Dorn, McGrath, and Holahan, "What Is the Result of States Not Expanding Medicaid?"

136. Lizette Alvarez and Christine Jordan Sexton, "Florida Runs Out of Time on Medicaid," *New York Times,* May 2, 2013, A11.

137. Alex Leary, "At CPAC, House Speaker Will Weatherford Emphasizes Opposition to Medicaid Expansion," *Miami Herald,* March 29, 2013, accessed November 14, 2014, http://www.miami herald.com/news/politics-government/article1948287.html.

138. Tia Mitchell, "Florida Chamber Endorses Medicaid Expansion—with Caveats," *Tampa Bay Times,* March 8, 2013, accessed November 14, 2014, http://www.tampabay.com/news/business /florida-chamber-endorses-medicaid-expansion-8212-with-caveats/2107928.

139. Thompson, *Medicaid Politics,* 193.

140. In March 2013, a poll conducted by the Associated Industries of Florida found support for the expansion running ahead of opposition by 54 percent to 31 percent. Interestingly the margins were significantly higher in the Latino community. In the 2012 election the Obama campaign, which largely steered away from talking about the ACA, did target Spanish-language advertisements at Latino communities. Marc Caputo, "Fight over Obamacare Is Anything but Over in Florida," *Kaiser Health News,* last modified September 24, 2013, accessed November 14, 2014, http://www.kaiserhealthnews.org/stories/2013/september/24/fight-over-obamacare-is-anything-but-over-in-florida.aspx.

141. Kliff, "Republican Governors Have Found Something They Like about Obamacare."

142. Kaiser Commission on Medicaid and the Uninsured, "Healthy Indiana Plan and the Affordable Care Act," last modified December 18, 2013, accessed November 14, 2014, http://kff.org/medicaid/fact-sheet/healthy-indiana-plan-and-the-affordable-care-act/.

143. On the Democrats and their opposition to health savings accounts, see Douglas Jaenicke and Alex Waddan, "President Bush and Social Policy: The Strange Case of the Medicare Prescription Drug Benefit," *Political Science Quarterly* 121, no. 2 (2006): 217–240.

144. Sarah Kliff, "A Bright 'Red Line': What the White House Won't Do to Woo GOP Governors into Obamacare," Vox.com, August 29, 2014, accessed November 14, 2014, http://www.vox.com/2014/8/29/6082841/a-bright-red-line-what-the-white-house-wont-do-to-woo-gop-governors.

145. Robert Pear, "Expanding Medicaid with Private Insurance," *New York Times,* March 22, 2013, A14.

146. Christine Vestal, "Ohio, Arkansas May Provide New Model for Insuring Low-Income Residents," *Kaiser Health News,* last modified March 22, 2013, accessed November 14, 2014, http://www.kaiserhealthnews.org/Stories/2013/March/22/medicaid-expansion-private-insurance-states.aspx.

147. Paul Waldman, "The Cruelty of Republican States in One Chart," *American Prospect,* last modified October 3, 2013, accessed November 14, 2014, http://prospect.org/article/cruelty-republican-states-one-chart.

148. By this projection, only Mississippi had a higher increase than Arkansas. This simulation assumed little so-called "woodwork effect." John Holahan and Irene Headen, *Medicaid Coverage and Spending in Health Reform: National and State by State Results for Adults at or Below 133% FPL* (Washington, DC: Kaiser Commission on Medicaid and the Uninsured, 2010), 10.

149. Robert Pear, "In Health Care Ruling, Vast Implications for Medicaid," *New York Times,* June 16, 2012, A12.

150. In regional terms, Arkansas had actually been something of a laggard in its switch from Democratic to GOP control. However, the 2012 results meant that the "historic switch of parties is now complete: 10 Deep South states have changed from total Democratic control to total Republican control." Dennis Cauchon, "Democrats Gain Ground in State Legislatures," *USA Today,* November 7, 2012, accessed November 14, 2014, http://www.usatoday.com/story/news/politics/2012/11/07/dems-gain-ground-in-state-legislatures/1690497/.

151. David Morgan, "Analysis: Arkansas Republicans Seek Acceptable 'Obamacare,'" Reuters, March 19, 2013, accessed November 14, 2014, http://www.reuters.com/article/2013/03/19/us-usa-healthcare-medicaid-idUSBRE92I0Y920130319.

152. Jesse Cross-Call and Judith Solomon, *Approved Demonstrations Offer Lessons for States Seeking to Expand Medicaid through Waivers,* Center on Budget and Policy Priorities, August 2014, accessed November 14, 2014, http://www.cbpp.org/files/8-20-14health.pdf.

153. Suzi Parker, "Arkansas Health Plan for Poor to Add Limited Federal Costs: Report," Reuters, March 18, 2013, accessed November 14, 2014, http://www.reuters.com/article/2013/03/19/us-medicaid-arkansas-idUSBRE92I02K20130319.

154. Morgan, "Analysis: Arkansas Republicans Seek Acceptable 'Obamacare.'"

155. State of Arkansas Bill 1145, accessed November 14, 2014, ftp://www.arkleg.state.ar.us/acts/2013/Public/ACT1498.pdf.

156. "Arkansas 1115 Waiver Application," August 2, 2013, accessed November 14, 2014, http://humanservices.arkansas.gov/dms/Documents/Final%201115%20Waiver%20Materials%20for%20Submission.pdf.

157. Robert Pear, "One State's Way to Bolster Health Coverage for the Poor," New York Times, September 27, 2013, accessed November 14, 2014, http://www.nytimes.com/news/affordable-care-act/2013/09/27/one-states-way-to-boost-health-coverage-for-poor/?_php=true&_type=blogs&_r=0.

158. Morgan, "Analysis: Arkansas Republicans Seek Acceptable 'Obamacare.'"

159. Jonathan Dismang, "The Private Option Is Leading to True Entitlement Reform," Talk Business and Politics, January 14, 2014, accessed November 14, 2014, http://talkbusiness.net/2014/01/sen-jonathan-dismang-private-option-leading-true-entitlement-reform/.

160. Nicole Kaeding, "The Arkansas Scheme to Expand Medicaid," Americans for Prosperity, last modified April 4, 2013, accessed November 14, 2014, http://americansforprosperity.org/legislativealerts/the-arkansas-scheme-to-expand-medicaid.

161. Nina Owcharenko, "Think Again: The Arkansas Plan for Medicaid Is Still a Bad Idea," Daily Signal, May 16, 2013, accessed November 14, 2014, http://dailysignal.com/2013/05/16/think-again-the-arkansas-plan-for-medicaid-is-still-a-bad-idea/.

162. Sophie Novack, "Arkansas Just Funded Its Medicaid Expansion—but the Fight Isn't Over," National Journal, March 4, 2014, accessed November 14, 2014, http://www.nationaljournal.com/health-care/arkansas-just-funded-its-medicaid-expansion-but-the-fight-isn-t-over-20140304.

5. REGULATORY REFORM

1. Kaiser Family Foundation, Health Insurance Reform: Rate Review, Publication 8392 (Menlo Park, CA: Kaiser Family Foundation, 2012); Kaiser Family Foundation, "Explaining Health Care Reform: Medical Loss Ratio," last modified February 29, 2012, accessed October 24, 2014, http://kff.org/health-reform/fact-sheet/explaining-health-care-reform-medical-loss-ratio-mlr/.

2. Quoted in Dan Managan, "Obamacare's $3 Billion Windfall to Insurance Customers," CNBC News, May 13, 2014, accessed October 24, 2014, http://www.cnbc.com/id/101665134.

3. Duke Helfland, "Blue Shield of California Defies State Insurance Commissioner on Rate Hikes," Los Angeles Times, January 14, 2011, accessed June 8, 2014, http://latimesblogs.latimes.com/money_co/2011/01/blue-shield-of-california-defies-state-insurance-commissioner-on-rate-hikes.html.

4. Ibid.

5. "Insurers Nervous over Prospect of Romney Victory," NewsOK.com, October 29, 2012, accessed June 8, 2014, http://newsok.com/insurers-nervous-over-prospect-of-romney-victory/article/feed/454451.

6. In addition to the medical loss ratio and rate review provisions (sec. 1001 and sec. 1003, respectively) discussed here, many core regulatory provisions can be found in the ACA's Subtitle C ("Quality Health Insurance Coverage for All Americans"), which includes preexisting condi-

tion exclusions, regulations on state geographical rating areas, guaranteed availability and renewability of coverage, prohibitions on health status discrimination, and prohibitions on excessive wait times.

7. Katie Keith and Kevin W. Lucia, "Implementing the Affordable Care Act: The State of the States," Commonwealth Fund, January 2014, http://www.commonwealthfund.org/~/media/Files /Publications/Fund%20Report/2014/Jan/1727_Keith_implementing_ACA_state_of_states.pdf.

8. Karen Pollitz, Nicole Tapay, Elizabeth Hadley, and Jalena Specht, "Early Experience with 'New Federalism' in Health Insurance Regulation," *Health Affairs* 19, no. 4 (2000): 7.

9. Keith and Lucia, "Implementing the Affordable Care Act."

10. Kaiser Family Foundation, *Health Insurance Reform.*

11. National Association of Insurance Commissioners, "Survey on State Authority to Enforce PPACA Immediate Implementation Provisions," August 5, 2010, accessed November 5, 2014, http://www.naic.org/documents/index_health_reform_section_ppaca_state_enforcement _authority.pdf.

12. Kaiser Family Foundation, *Health Insurance Reform.*

13. Centers for Medicare and Medicaid Services, "Rate Increase Disclosure and Review: Final Rule, CMS-9999-FC," accessed June 7, 2014, http://www.kyequaljustice.org/file/history/KEJC -CMS-9999-FC.pdf.

14. Patient Protection and Affordable Care Act, Public Law 111-148, sec. 1003.

15. Ibid., sec. 1001; see also Mark Hall and Michael McCue, "Estimating the Impact of the Medical Loss Ratio Rule: A State-by-State Analysis," Commonwealth Fund, April 2012, accessed June 12, 2014, http://www.commonwealthfund.org/~/media/files/publications/issue-brief/2012 /mar/1587_hall_medical_loss_ratio_ib.pdf.

16. Senate Committee on Commerce, Science, and Transportation, "Majority Staff Report on Implementing Health Insurance Reform: New Medical Loss Ratio Information for Policymakers and Consumers," April 15, 2010.

17. Patient Protection and Affordable Care Act, sec. 1001.

18. Ibid.

19. Ibid.

20. Centers for Medicare and Medicaid Services, "State Requests for MLR Adjustment," accessed June 27, 2014, http://www.cms.gov/CCIIO/Programs-and-Initiatives/Health-Insurance -Market-Reforms/state_mlr_adj_requests.html.

21. Susan Randall, "Insurance Regulation in the United States: Regulatory Federalism and the National Association of Insurance Commissioners," *Florida State University Law Review* 26 (1998): 625.

22. Ibid.

23. Ibid.

24. Ibid.

25. Ibid.; consumer representative at National Association of Insurance Commissioners (NAIC), interview by Philip Rocco, August 6, 2014.

26. Kaiser Family Foundation, "Rate Review: Spotlight on State Efforts to Make Healthcare More Affordable," December 2010, accessed June 14, 2014, http://thehill.com/images/stories /blogs/kaiser%20state.pdf.

27. Families USA, *Medical Loss Ratios: Evidence from the States* (Washington, DC: Families USA, June 2008).

28. Ibid.; Senate Committee on Commerce, Science, and Transportation, "Majority Staff Report on Implementing Health Insurance Reform."

29. Kaiser Family Foundation, "Rate Review."

30. Patient Protection and Affordable Care Act, sec. 1001 and 1003.

31. John Reichard, "Sebelius Shuffles Insurance Oversight Office into CMS, Shifts CLASS Act to Administration on Aging," *CQ HealthBeat,* last modified January 5, 2011, http://www.common wealthfund.org/publications/newsletters/washington-health-policy-in-review/2011/jan/january -10-2011/sebelius-shuffles-insurance-oversight-office.

32. Ibid.

33. Ibid.

34. Patient Protection and Affordable Care Act, sec. 1001.

35. Jean M. Abraham and Pinar Karaca-Mandic, "Regulating the Medical Loss Ratio: Implications for the Individual Market," *American Journal of Managed Care* 17, no. 3 (2011): 212.

36. Patient Protection and Affordable Care Act, sec. 1003.

37. Stephanie Condon, "Can Obama's Health Care Law Survive without the Individual Mandate?" *CBS News,* March 27, 2012, accessed June 20, 2014, http://www.cbsnews.com/news/can -obamas-health-care-law-survive-without-the-individual-mandate/.

38. Kaiser Family Foundation, Health Tracking Poll, February 29–March 5, 2012, accessed July 5, 2014, http://kff.org/health-reform/poll-finding/kaiser-health-tracking-poll-march-2012/.

39. On symbolic politics, see Timothy J. Conlan, Paul L. Posner, and David R. Beam, *Pathways of Power: The Dynamics of National Policymaking* (Washington, DC: Georgetown University Press, 2014): 89–105.

40. Federal official, interview by Philip Rocco and Daniel Béland, August 28, 2014.

41. Ibid.; federal official, interview by Philip Rocco, September 12, 2014.

42. State health insurance administrators, surveyed online by Philip Rocco, November 5, 2012–January 15, 2013.

43. Federal official, interview by Rocco.

44. Federal official, interview by Rocco and Béland.

45. State health insurance administrators, survey by Rocco.

46. Department of Health and Human Services, "Premium Review Process, Request for Comments Regarding Section 2794 of the Public Health Service Act, 75 FR 19335," April 14, 2010, accessed June 10, 2014, http://www.gpo.gov/fdsys/pkg/FR-2010-04-14/html/2010-8600.htm.

47. Insurance industry lobbyists to members of the NAIC, letters; see, for example, Karen Ignani to Kathleen Sebelius, letter, March 3, 2010, accessed June 15, 2014, http://www.ahip coverage.com/2010/03/04/ahips-letter-to-secretary-sebelius/. For a combined set of industry comments for the NAIC's rate review and MLR deliberations, see http://www.naic.org/documents /committees_e_hrsi_comments_0512exposure_combined.pdf.

48. America's Health Insurance Plans (AHIP) to the Department of Health and Human Services (HHS), letters, spring 2010; for example, Jeffrey Gabardi to Donald Moulds, letter, May 14, 2010, accessed October 1, 2014, http://www.ahip.org/Issues/Documents/2010/AHIP-Letter-to -HHS-on-Health-Insurance-Rate-Review.aspx.

49. National Association of Insurance Commissioners (NAIC), "Response to Request for Information Regarding Section 2794 of the Public Health Service Act," May 12, 2010.

50. Julie Appleby, "Insurance Regulators Wrestle with Definition of 'Unreasonable' Rate Increases," *Kaiser Health News,* last modified May 17, 2010, accessed March 12, 2014, http://www .kaiserhealthnews.org/Stories/2010/May/14/insurance-regulators-wrestle-with-definition-of -unreasonable-rate-increases.aspx?p=1.

51. Bill Weller and Cindy Gallaher to Lou Felice, letter, May 24, 2010, accessed March 12, 2014, http://www.naic.org/documents/committees_e_hrsi_comments_0520exposure_ahip_100524.pdf.

52. National Association of Insurance Commissioners (NAIC), "Rate Filing Disclosure Form," December 2010, accessed July 11, 2014, http://www.naic.org/documents/committees_exec _plenary_101216_rate_filing_form.pdf

53. Ibid.

54. Department of Health and Human Services, "Rate Increase Disclosure and Review, Notice of Proposed Rulemaking, OCIIO-9999-P," 17–18, accessed July 15, 2014, http://thehill.com /images/stories/blogs/ratereview.pdf.

55. Ibid., 18–19.

56. Ibid., 45.

57. Ibid., 20.

58. Ibid., 46.

59. Ibid.

60. Centers for Medicare and Medicaid Services (CMS), "State Effective Rate Review Programs," accessed October 27, 2014, http://www.cms.gov/CCIIO/Resources/Fact-Sheets-and -FAQs/rate_review_fact_sheet.html.

61. Timothy Jost, "Implementing Health Reform: Medical Loss Ratios," *Health Affairs Blog*, November 23, 2010, accessed October 12, 2104, http://healthaffairs.org/blog/2010/11/23/implement ing-health-reform-medical-loss-ratios/.

62. Ibid.

63. Consumer representative from NAIC, interview by Rocco.

64. National Association of Insurance Commissioners (NAIC), "Combined Comment Letters on Medical Loss Ratio Working Group," May 17, 2010, accessed August 12, 2014, http://www .naic.org/documents/committees_e_hrsi_comments_0512exposure_combined.pdf.

65. Joan McCarter, "Rockefeller: Time for Insurance Companies to Spend Money on Actual Care," *DailyKos*, October 1, 2009, accessed July 11, 2014, http://www.dailykos.com/story/2009 /10/01/788513/-Rockefeller-time-for-insurance-companies-to-spend-money-on-actual-care.

66. John D. Rockefeller to Kathleen Sebelius, letter, May 7, 2010; John D. Rockefeller to Jane Cline, letter, May 7, 2010.

67. Rockefeller to Sebelius, May 7, 2010.

68. Rockefeller to Cline, May 7, 2010.

69. This definition was ultimately used by the federal government. See Centers for Medicare and Medicaid Services (CMS), "Medical Loss Ratio (MLR), Annual Reporting Form Filing Instructions for the 2013 MLR Reporting Year," March 26, 2014.

70. John D. Rockefeller to Jane Cline, letter, October 14, 2010.

71. National Association of Insurance Commissioners (NAIC) to Kathleen Sebelius, letter, October 27, 2010.

72. Department of Health and Human Services, "Health Insurance Issuers Implementing Medical Loss Ratio (MLR) Requirements under the Patient Protection and Affordable Care Act, 75 Fed. Reg. 74875," December 1, 2010.

73. Senate Committee on Commerce, Science, and Transportation, "Majority Staff Report on Consumer Health Insurance Savings under the Medical Loss Ratio Law," May 24, 2011.

74. Michael D. Maves to Kathleen Sebelius, letter, January 31, 2011.

75. Ken A. Crerar to the Office of Consumer Information and Insurance Oversight, letter, January 31, 2011; Janet Trautwein to Kathleen Sebelius, letter, January 28, 2011.

76. Randel K. Johnson and Katie Mahoney to the Office of Consumer Information and Insurance Oversight, letter, January 31, 2011.

77. NAIC consumer representative, interview by Philip Rocco, August 6, 2014.

78. Sean P. Carr, "NAIC Picks New Leaders in Wake of Electoral Defeat," *InsuranceNews.net,* December 15, 2010, accessed August 8, 2014, http://insurancenewsnet.com/oarticle/2010/12/15 /naic-picks-new-leaders-in-wake-of-electoral-defeat-a-240090.html#.U3UZvcfBre8.

79. Arthur D. Postal, "Rockefeller Objects to MLR Agent Exemption; NAIC to Hold Hearing," *PropertyCasualty360,* last modified March 16, 2011, accessed June 14, 2014, http://www.property casualty360.com/2011/03/16/rockefeller-objects-to-mlr-agent-exemption-naic-to.

80. Arthur D. Postal, "NAIC Panel Seeks More Info before Backing Agent MLR Exemption," *Consumer Watchdog,* March 28, 2011.

81. Senate Committee on Commerce, Science, and Transportation, "Majority Staff Report on Consumer Health Insurance Savings under the Medical Loss Ratio Law."

82. Postal, "NAIC Panel Seeks More Info before Backing Agent MLR Exemption."

83. Elizabeth D. Festa, "NAIC Narrowly Passes Resolution Urging HHS to Exempt Agent Commissions from PPACA Standard," *LifeHealthPro,* last modified November 22, 2011, accessed October 14, 2014, http://www.lifehealthpro.com/2011/11/22/naic-narrowly-passes-resolution -urging-hhs-to-exem?page=3.

84. Ibid.

85. Department of Health and Human Services, "Medical Loss Ratio Requirements under the Patient Protection and Affordable Care Act, CMS-9998-FC," December 7, 2011.

86. Ibid.

87. Department of Health and Human Services, "Medical Loss Ratio Requirements under the Patient Protection and Affordable Care Act, CMS-9998-F," last modified May 16, 2012, http:// www.gpo.gov/fdsys/pkg/FR-2012-05-16/pdf/2012-11753.pdf; CMS-9998-IFC3; Medical Loss Ratio Requirements under the Patient Protection and Affordable Care Act, Correcting Amendment, May 16, 2012, http://www.gpo.gov/fdsys/pkg/FR-2012-05-16/pdf/2012–11773.pdf.

88. US Government Accountability Office (GAO), "Early Indicators Show That Most Insurers Would Have Met or Exceeded New Medical Loss Ratio Standards, GAO-12-90R," last modified October 31, 2011, accessed October 20, 2014, http://www.gao.gov/products/GAO-12-90R.

89. John Barven, "More Action around MLR (Medical Loss Ratio) Requirements," Benico .com, last modified May 24, 2011, accessed October 20, 2014, http://benico.com/2011/05/more -action-around-mlr-medical-loss-ratio-requirements-nahu-post/.

90. Texas Department of Insurance, "Request for Adjustment to the Medical Loss Ratio," accessed October 4, 2014, http://cciio.cms.gov/programs/marketreforms/mlr/states/texas/tx_mlr _adj_request_07292011.pdf.

91. Ibid.

92. Steven Larsen to Eleanor Kitzman, letter, January 27, 2012, accessed July 2, 2014, http:// www.cms.gov/CCIIO/Programs-and-Initiatives/Health-Insurance-Market-Reforms/Down loads/012712_FINAL_TX_MLR_Adj_Determination_Letter.pdf.

93. Ibid.

94. Ibid.

95. Ibid.

96. Jane Norman, "Kaiser Study Projects $1.4 Billion in Medical Loss Ratio Rebates," *CQ Health Beat,* last modified April 30, 2012.

97. Public Act 11-58, HB 6308.

98. Connecticut General Assembly, "Substitute Raised for H.B. No. 6308, Session Year 2011," accessed October 24, 2014, http://www.cga.ct.gov/asp/cgabillstatus/cgabillstatus.asp ?selBillType=Bill&bill_num=HB06308&which_year=2011.

99. Dannel Molloy to Denise W. Merrill, letter, July 1, 2011.

100. This conclusion is based on analysis of Center for Consumer Information and Insurance Oversight, "Rate Review Data," accessed June 7, 2014, http://www.cms.gov/CCIIO/Resources/Data-Resources/ratereview.html.

101. Arielle Levin Becker, "After Rate Hike Rejected, Anthem to Decrease Premiums Next Year," *CT Mirror*, August 15, 2014, accessed October 24, 2014, http://ctmirror.org/after-rate-hike-rejected-anthem-to-decrease-premiums-next-year/.

102. Sam Stein, "Mitch Daniels Not Only Took ObamaCare Funds, He Pushed Similar Reforms," *Huffington Post*, May 19, 2011, accessed October 21, 2014, http://www.huffingtonpost.com/2011/05/19/mitch-daniels-obamacare-similar-reforms_n_864157.html.

103. Michael F. Cannon, "Mitch Daniels's Obamacare Problem," *National Review*, March 4, 2011, accessed October 21, 2014, http://www.nationalreview.com/articles/261285/mitch-daniels-s-obamacare-problem-michael-f-cannon.

104. Katie Keith, Kevin Lucia, and Sabrina Corlette, "Implementing the Affordable Care Act: State Action on Early Market Reforms," Commonwealth Fund, last modified March 2012, accessed September 10, 2014, http://www.commonwealthfund.org/publications/issue-briefs/2012/mar/state-action.

105. Indiana General Assembly, Senate Bill 461, last modified April 12, 2011, accessed October 20, 2014, http://www.in.gov/legislative/bills/2011/ES/ES0461.2.html.

106. Indiana General Assembly, Senate motion, last modified April 14, 2011, accessed October 25, 2014, http://www.in.gov/legislative/bills/2011/SAMP/RS046101.D.html.

107. Indiana General Assembly, Senate Enrolled Act 461, accessed October 2, 2014, http://www.in.gov/legislative/bills/2011/SE/SE0461.1.html.

108. Indiana General Assembly, Action List, Senate Bill 461, accessed October 25, 2014, http://www.in.gov/apps/lsa/session/billwatch/billinfo?year=2011&request=getActions&doctype=SB&docno=0461.

109. Indiana Department of Insurance, press release, June 1, 2011, accessed November 1, 2014, www.in.gov/idoi/files/Rate_Review_Press_Release.pdf; Stephen W. Robertson to Kathleen Sebelius, letter, May 27, 2011, accessed November 1, 2014, www.kokomoherald.com/FTP/Sebelius%20Letter.pdf.

110. Assistant Secretary for Planning and Evaluation, "Annual Rate Review Report: 2013," accessed July 15, 2014, http://aspe.hhs.gov/health/reports/2013/acaannualreport/ratereview_rpt.cfm.

111. American Legislative Exchange Council, *The State Legislators Guide to Repealing Obama-Care* (Washington, DC: ALEC, 2011), 9.

112. Ibid., 13–15.

113. Ibid., 15.

114. National Conference of State Legislatures, "26 States Consider Health Compacts to Challenge Federal PPACA," last modified May 31, 2014, accessed October 27, 2014, http://www.ncsl.org/research/health/states-pursue-health-compacts.aspx.

115. Jim Ridling, "Affordable Care Act Form Filing Requirements," *Bulletin 2013-05*, April 17, 2013.

116. Rockefeller Institute, *Alabama: Round 1, State Level Field Network Study of the Implementation of the Affordable Care Act* (Albany, NY: Rockefeller Institute, 2014); Rockefeller Institute, *Texas: Round 1, State Level Field Network Study of the Implementation of the Affordable Care Act* (Albany, NY: Rockefeller Institute, 2014); Shefali Luthra, "State to Feds: We Won't Enforce Insurance Reforms," *Texas Tribune*, August 7, 2013, accessed October 4, 2014, http://www.texastribune.org/2013/08/07/state-not-enforce-key-health-reforms/.

117. Georgia Senate Bill 22, introduced January 26, 2011.

118. New Jersey Assembly Bill 1674, introduced January 12, 2010.

119. This conclusion is based on searches of state legislation in LexisNexis and in the National Conference of State Legislatures (NCSL) Health Reform Legislative Tracking Database.

120. Tennessee Senate Bill 2155, passed April 10, 2014, accessed June 24, 2014, http://open states.org/tn/bills/108/SB2155/.

121. Keith, Lucia, and Corlette, "Implementing the Affordable Care Act."

122. Patient Protection and Affordable Care Act, sec. 1003.

123. US Government Accountability Office (GAO), "Patient Protection and Affordable Care Act: HHS's Process for Awarding and Overseeing Exchange and Rate Review Grants to States, GAO-15-543," last modified May 31, 2013, accessed June 24, 2014, http://www.gao.gov/products /GAO-13-543.

124. Ibid.

125. Ibid.; Igor Volsky, "19 of the 22 States Suing Government over Health Reform Willing to Accept Grant Money from Law," *Think Progress*, last modified August 16, 2010, accessed June 20, 2014, http://thinkprogress.org/health/2010/08/16/171597/rate-review-repeal/.

126. American Legislative Exchange Council, *State Legislators Guide to Repealing Obama-Care*, 13–15.

127. GAO, "Patient Protection and Affordable Care Act," 46; Margie Manning, "Reform Limbo: Florida Rejects Money for Rate-Hike Review," *Tampa Bay Business Journal*, March 31, 2011, accessed August 12, 2014, http://www.bizjournals.com/tampabay/print-edition/2011/04/01 /reform-limbo-florida-rejects-money.html?page=all.

128. John Huff, "Patient Protection and Affordable Care Act Policy Filing Guidelines," *Insurance Bulletin 10-05*, September 23, 2010, accessed November 2, 2014, https://insurance.mo.gov / . . . /InsuranceBulletin10-05.pdf.

129. Samantha Liss, "Missouri Lags Behind in Insurance Pricing Transparency," *St. Louis Post-Dispatch*, August 18, 2014, accessed October 24, 2014, http://kaiserhealthnews.org/news /missouri-lags-behind-in-insurance-pricing-transparency/; Centers for Medicare and Medicaid Services, "Missouri Rate Review Grant Awards List," accessed October 27, 2014, http://www.cms .gov/cciio/Resources/Rate-Review-Grants/mo.html.

130. Denny Hoskins, "Hoskins: 'Full Steam Ahead' on HB45, Committee Updates," *Missives from Missouri*, January 21, 2011, accessed October 27, 2014, http://missivesfrommo.blogspot .com/2011/01/hoskins-full-steam-ahead-on-hb45.html.

131. Missouri House of Representatives, "Activity History for HB 45," accessed October 26, 2014, http://www.house.mo.gov/BillActions.aspx?bill=HB45&year=2011&code=R.

132. Chris Blank, "Missouri Lawmakers Approve Bill to Aid Small Businesses," NewsTribune .com, May 1, 2011, accessed October 27, 2014, http://www.newstribune.com/news/2011/may/01 /missouri-lawmakers-approve-bill-aid-small-business/.

133. GAO, "Patient Protection and Affordable Care Act."

134. Keith, Lucia, and Corlette, "Implementing the Affordable Care Act."

135. Janice K. Brewer, veto message on Senate Bill 1592, April 18, 2011, accessed November 9, 2014, http://www.kpho.com/download/2011/0419/27599536.pdf.

136. Ibid.

137. Ibid.

138. "Votes AZ HB 2550, 2013, Fifty-First Legislature 1st Regular," LegiScan, accessed October 26, 2014, http://legiscan.com/AZ/votes/HB2550/2013.

139. Keith, Lucia, and Corlette, "Implementing the Affordable Care Act."

140. Ibid.

141. Arizona Department of Insurance, "Health Insurance: Rate Review Grant," accessed October 26, 2014, http://www.azinsurance.gov/RateReview/index.html.

142. Ibid.

143. CMS, "State Effective Rate Review Programs."

144. Germaine Marks, "Threshold Rate Increase Review," *Regulatory Bulletin 201244*, December 21, 2012, accessed November 9, 2014, www.azinsurance.gov/bulletin/2012-04.pdf.

145. Jacob S. Hacker, "Privatizing Risk without Privatizing the Welfare State: The Hidden Politics of Social Policy Retrenchment in the United States," *American Political Science Review* 98, no. 2 (2004): 244.

146. For discussion of the impact of varying rate review programs, see Kaiser Family Foundation, "Quantifying the Effects of Health Insurance Rate Review," last modified October 1, 2012, http://kff.org/health-costs/report/quantifying-the-effects-of-health-insurance-rate/.

147. Ibid., 9.

148. NORC, University of Chicago, *Effects of Implementing State Insurance Market Reform, 2011–2012* (Chicago: NORC, 2013), 63.

149. Sabrina Corlette, Christine Monahan, and Kevin Lucia, "Moving to High Quality, Adequate Coverage: State Implementation of New Essential Health Benefit Requirements," Robert Wood Johnson Foundation Report, last modified August 2013, accessed August 19, 2014, http://www.rwjf.org/en/research-publications/find-rwjf-research/2013/08/moving-to-high-quality-adequate-coverage-state-implementation.html.

150. Urban Institute, "Health Reform Monitoring Study, Quarter 3," 2013, accessed October 24, 2014, http://hrms.urban.org/briefs/awareness-of-provision.html.

151. Patient Protection and Affordable Care Act, sec. 1002.

152. Natalie Villacorta, "Who Will Help the Newly Insured?" *Politico*, February 18, 2104, accessed October 26, 2014, http://www.politico.com/story/2014/02/obamacare-newly-insured-103645.html.

153. Kaiser Family Foundation, Karen Pollitz, Jennifer Tolbert, and Rosa Ma, "Survey of Health Insurance Marketplace Assister Programs," last modified June 15, 2014, accessed October 12, 2014, http://kff.org/health-reform/report/survey-of-health-insurance-marketplace-assister-programs/.

CONCLUSION

1. Eric M. Patashnik, *Reforms at Risk: What Happens after Major Policy Changes Are Enacted* (Princeton, NJ: Princeton University Press, 2008).

2. See Eric M. Patashnik and Julian E. Zelizer, "The Struggle to Remake Politics: Liberal Reform and the Limits of Policy Feedback in the Contemporary American State," *Perspectives on Politics* 11, no. 4 (2013): 1071–1087. See also Vesla Weaver, "The Significance of Policy Failures in Political Development: The Law Enforcement Assistance Administration in the Carceral State," in *Living Legislation: Durability, Change, and the Politics of American Lawmaking*, ed. Jeffrey Jenkins and Eric M. Patashnik (Chicago: University of Chicago Press, 2012), 221–254.

3. Frank J. Thompson, *Medicaid Politics: Federalism, Policy Durability, and Health Reform* (Washington, DC: Georgetown University Press, 2012).

4. Herbert Obinger, Stephan Leibfried, and Frank G. Castles, eds., *Federalism and the Welfare State: New World and European Experiences* (Cambridge, UK: Cambridge University Press,

2005). A good example of this concerns the way fiscal horizontal redistribution operates in these three countries; see Daniel Béland and André Lecours, "Accommodation and the Politics of Fiscal Equalization in Multinational States: The Case of Canada," *Nations and Nationalism* 20, no. 2 (2014): 337–354.

5. On differences in the politics of federalism within the same country between different social programs, see Keith G. Banting, "Canada: Nation-Building in a Federal Welfare State," in *Federalism and the Welfare State: New World and European Experiences,* ed. Herbert Obinger, Stephan Leibfried, and Frank G. Castles (Cambridge, UK: Cambridge University Press, 2005), 89–137; Daniel Béland and John Myles, "Varieties of Federalism, Institutional Legacies, and Social Policy: Comparing Old-Age and Unemployment Insurance Reform in Canada," *International Journal of Social Welfare* 21, no. S1 (2012): S75–S87.

6. John Dinan, "Contemporary Assertions of State Sovereignty and the Safeguards of American Federalism," *Albany Law Review* 74 (2010): 1635–1667.

7. Christine Vestal, "Court Rulings Add Urgency to State Exchange Decisions," PEW Charitable Trusts, last modified August 4, 2014, accessed August 31, 2014, http://www.pewtrusts.org /en/research-and-analysis/blogs/stateline/2014/08/04/court-rulings-add-urgency-to-state -exchange-decisions.

8. *King v. Burwell,* 576 U.S. ___ (2015).

9. Stuart M. Butler, "Why the GOP Needs an Alternative to the Obamacare Repeal Strategy," *Health360,* January 28, 2015, accessed June 12, 2015, http://www.brookings.edu/blogs/health360 /posts/2015/01/28-gop-obamacare-repeal-strategy-alternative-butler.

10. Deborah Bachrach, Joel Ario, and Hailey Davis, *Innovation Waivers: An Opportunity for States to Pursue Their Own Brand of Health Reform,* Commonwealth Fund/Robert Wood Johnson Foundation, April 2015.

11. Stan Dorn, Megan McGrath, and John Holahan, "What Is the Result of States Not Expanding Medicaid?" Robert Wood Johnson Foundation/Urban Institute, accessed October 24, 2014, http://www.rwjf.org/content/dam/farm/reports/issue_briefs/2014/rwjf414946.

12. Andrew Kitchenman, "ACA Provision Returns Billions to Consumers, Harkens Back to NJ Reforms of the Early 1990s," *NJ Spotlight,* July 27, 2014, accessed July 28, 2014, http://www .njspotlight.com/stories/14/07/27/aca-provision-returns-billions-to-consumers-harkens-back -to-nj-reforms-of-early-1990s/.

13. Allison Bell, "MLR Rebate Total Falls Again," *Life Health Pro,* July 24, 2014, accessed July 24, 2014, http://www.lifehealthpro.com/2014/07/24/hhs-mlr-rebate-total-falls-again.

14. US Government Accountability Office (GAO), *Early Effects of Medical Loss Ratio Requirements and Rebates on Insurers and Enrollees,* GAO-14-580 (Washington, DC: Government Printing Office, 2014).

15. Kaiser Family Foundation, "Rate Review Processes in the Individual and Group Markets," accessed August 31, 2014, http://kff.org/health-reform/state-indicator/rate-review-program -effectiveness/.

16. "Voters Defeat Health Insurance Rate Initiative," November 4, 2014, http://www.news10 .net/story/news/local/california/2014/11/05/california-election-results-for-prop-45/18512765/#; "Covered California Questions Rate Review Ballot Initiative," KQED, June 19, 2014, accessed June 19, 2014, http://www.californiahealthline.org/articles/2014/6/19/covered-california-questions -rate-review-ballot-initiative.

17. For a discussion of some of these issues, see Scott E. Harrington and Janet Weiner, *Deciphering the Data: Health Insurance Rates and Rate Review* (Philadelphia: Leonard Davis Institute of Health Economics/Robert Wood Johnson Foundation, 2014).

18. "2014 Governor Election Results," *New York Times,* accessed November 18, 2014, http:// elections.nytimes.com/2014/results/governor; "State Legislative Elections, 2014," *Ballotpedia,* accessed November 18, 2014, http://ballotpedia.org/State_legislative_elections,_2014.

19. John Wagner and Jenna Johnson, "Republican Larry Hogan Wins Md. Governor's Race in Stunning Upset," *Washington Post,* November 5, 2014, accessed November 5, 2014, http://www .washingtonpost.com/local/md-politics/republican-larry-hogan-wins-md-governors-race-in -stunning-upset/2014/11/05/9eb8bf46-60ac-11e4-8b9e-2ccdac31a031_story.html.

20. Liz Farmer, "Arizona Votes for Opting Out of Federal Laws," *Governing,* November 5, accessed November 5, 2014, http://www.governing.com/topics/elections/gov-arizona-federal-laws -ballot.html.

21. Kaiser Family Foundation, "Health Tracking Poll: Exploring the Public's Views on the Affordable Care Act," accessed August 31, 2014, http://kff.org/interactive/health-tracking-poll -exploring-the-publics-views-on-the-affordable-care-act-aca/.

INDEX

Printed in the USA
CPSIA information can be obtained
at www.ICGtesting.com
CBHW061302060524
8104CB00006B/784